THE PRACTICE OF SHIATSU

D0565513

THE PRACTICE OF SHIATSU

Sandra K. Anderson, BA, LMT, NCTMB
Co-Owner, Tucson Touch Therapies
Treatment Center and Education Center
Tucson, Arizona

With 355 full-color illustrations

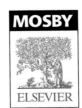

MOSBY

ELSEVIER

11830 Westline Industrial Drive
St. Louis, Missouri 63146

THE PRACTICE OF SHIATSU

ISBN: 978-0-323-04580-3

Copyright © 2008 by Mosby, Inc., an affiliate of Elsevier Inc.

All rights reserved. No part of this publication may be reproduced or transmitted in any form or by any means, electronic or mechanical, including photocopying, recording, or any information storage and retrieval system, without permission in writing from the publisher.
Permissions may be sought directly from Elsevier's Health Sciences Rights Department in Philadelphia, PA, USA: phone: (+1) 215 239 3804, fax: (+1) 215 239 3805, e-mail: healthpermissions@elsevier.com. You may also complete your request on-line via the Elsevier homepage (http://www.elsevier.com), by selecting "Customer Support" and then "Obtaining Permissions."

Notice

Neither the Publisher nor the Author assumes any responsibility for any loss or injury and/or damage to persons or property arising out of or related to any use of the material contained in this book. It is the responsibility of the treating practitioner, relying on independent expertise and knowledge of the patient, to determine the best treatment and method of application for the patient.

The Publisher

Library of Congress Control Number: 2007928476

Publishing Director: Linda Duncan
Senior Editor: Kellie White
Senior Developmental Editor: Jennifer Watrous
Publishing Services Manager: Patricia Tannian
Project Manager: Claire Kramer
Book Designer: Kimberly E. Denando

Working together to grow
libraries in developing countries

www.elsevier.com | www.bookaid.org | www.sabre.org

ELSEVIER | BOOK AID International | Sabre Foundation

Printed in China

Last digit is the print number: 9 8 7 6 5 4 3 2 1

To David Kent Anderson, who knows all the reasons why

To my sisters, Sue Kauffman and Linda Kauffman Guenther: two beautiful, lively, and intelligent women who help make life wonderful

CONTRIBUTORS

Tama Hader, NCBTMB
Certification, Zen Shiatsu
Certification, Thai Massage
Private Practice, Listening Hands Shiatsu
Columbia Falls, Montana
Contributions Throughout the Book

Cora Jacobson
Owner, Touch of Radiance Healing Arts
Tucson, Arizona
Chapter 8

Bob Lehnberg
Certified Teacher of Body-Mind Centering © and Qigong
Lewisville, North Carolina
Qigong Section, Chapter 5

REVIEWERS

William Courtland, LMT, AS, NCTMB
Faculty Member
Acupressure and Chinese Medical Therapy
Connecticut Center for Massage Therapy
Westport, Connecticut

Jeanne deMontagnac-Hall, LMT, ABMP
Member, Massage Therapy Advisory Committee, Ohio
Member, Ohio Association of Blood Banks, Ohio
West Chester, Ohio

Eric Munn, CMT
Massage Therapy Program Director
Berdan Institute
Wayne, New Jersey

Terry Norman, BME, LMT, NCBTMB, AOBTA
Instructor
Texas Christian University
Tarrant County College So. Campus
University of Texas at Arlington
Mt. View Community College
Private Practice
Mansfield, Texas

FOREWORD

Shiatsu is a bodywork modality with roots in traditional Chinese medicine, various forms of Japanese massage, and a Western understanding of anatomy and physiology. In fact, shiatsu is the perfect meeting of Eastern and Western approaches to the human body. Its power lies in its approach to assessment and treatment. Shiatsu takes the whole person into consideration—the client's mental, emotional, and physical state—and seeks to restore harmony and balance.

Western science is gradually accepting, if somewhat grudgingly, the notion of mind-body interconnectedness (e.g., see *Molecules of Emotion: The Science Behind Mind-Body Medicine*, by Candace Pert, PhD). Not surprisingly (given its Asian roots), the concept of interconnectedness is inherent in shiatsu. The Western physiology term is *homeostasis,* and we learn in physiology class that the body is always seeking homeostasis. It literally means "same state" and refers to the process of keeping the internal body environment in a steady state of equilibrium. The importance of this cannot be overstressed because "internal body environment" includes our mental and emotional states. A great deal of the hormone system and autonomic nervous system is dedicated to homeostasis. Symptoms occur when homeostasis is disturbed, through injury, illness, or stress. Shiatsu has proved to be an effective modality for supporting the body in restoring overall homeostasis.

Shiatsu is now part of the curriculum at a large number of massage schools all over the country, and you can pick up books on shiatsu at most bookstores. The shiatsu books available either are aimed at a general audience (e.g., do-it-yourself shiatsu, treat your family and friends with shiatsu) or are more suitable for acupuncture students (i.e., they are considerably more technical and involved than a shiatsu practitioner needs).

The massage school I went to offered an evening program that combined massage certification with shiatsu training. I was excited about learning both Western and Eastern modalities. However, there was many a night when studying Western physiology and pathology alongside traditional Chinese medicine and Five Element Theory made my brain go *TILT.** Although the textbooks that were used for shiatsu were of good quality, they amounted to overkill—dizzyingly complex.

Fortunately, one of my shiatsu teachers was Sandy Anderson.

Sandy is an eminently practical person. As a teacher, she was able to translate an Eastern worldview and abstract concepts into language and exercises that made sense to us Western-schooled students. Now, as a writer, Sandy has produced a book that fills a big gap in shiatsu education. Through her review of the literature and her experience as both a practitioner and teacher of shiatsu, Sandy has crafted a book that provides the essential foundation to begin a practice of shiatsu.

When I was a student, the hardest concept for me to transfer from theory to practice was that of *Ki* (Japanese), or *Qi* (Chinese), which is variously translated as "energy" or "life force." Although I accepted the idea of Ki moving in channels (meridians) in the body, actually experiencing it and then applying the various theories (e.g., Yin/Yang, Five Element) were mind-bending challenges. In this book, Sandy effectively makes that bridge between theory and practice.

Sandy approaches the discussion of Ki by stressing the importance of connection—that shiatsu treatment happens as a result of the *connection* between practitioner and client—another aspect of the interconnectedness that pervades life. Because the quality of treatment is directly dependent on the quality of the connection between practitioner and client, Sandy provides the student with a variety of techniques to achieve a clear, open state.

In fact, one of the many strengths of the book is the emphasis on preparation. American culture is fast paced, and Americans are impatient for results. We take the fewest number of vacation days compared with any other country in the developed world. We

---

*I am of the generation that remembers pinball machines. Like the video games of today, they demanded good eye-hand coordination. Unlike today's electronic games, though, pinball machines are mechanical, and you could nudge the machine to help the ball move where you wanted it to go. If too much "body English" was used, though, the bumpers quit responding and the word *TILT* would appear in big, bright, flashing letters on the scoreboard. Game over.

must be constantly entertained, from television to music players to cell phones. As a culture, we do not recognize the value of being still. However, learning to be still is a prerequisite to sensing Ki and practicing shiatsu. This book provides clear guidance for learning this valuable skill through a framework of explanation and exercises that make it possible for a student to experience Ki, and to distinguish qualities of Ki, and then to find guidance for treating any disharmony or imbalance.

As any musician knows, perfecting basic scales is critical to later virtuosity. Sandy presents a basic *kata* (routine) to practice. Like practicing scales or committing a piece of music to memory, practicing a kata until it is part of you (e.g., not having to think about where to position yourself or how to move the client for access to a particular meridian) allows for total focus and openness to sensing the client's Ki and responding therapeutically.

Because of her considerable experience, Sandy emphasizes training her students in client-centered treatment. This means that students are encouraged to move beyond the basic routines, incorporating everything they have learned and experienced into a personal style that is uniquely responsive to each client they treat. For students learning shiatsu, this book provides a clear, measured path to that kind of virtuosity.

One of the things I most admire about Sandy is her passion for education. She is a marvelously effective teacher, with a love for the practice of shiatsu. She has experienced its therapeutic value firsthand from years of both giving and receiving shiatsu treatment. All that passion, knowledge, and experience have been channeled into this book—for you.

From foundational information to exercises to routines, from standard treatment protocols to methods of assessment and beyond, this book will guide you to that perfect marriage of education and experience that will make you an effective shiatsu practitioner. Many, many blessings for your journey.

Michaela Johnson, LMT
Massage therapist and shiatsu practitioner
Tucson, Arizona
March 2007

PREFACE

Shiatsu is a unique form of bodywork. It requires no special tools, lubricants, or equipment. It can be performed virtually anywhere. When shiatsu is done properly, both the practitioner and the recipient feel calm, balanced, and energized afterward. With its roots in the ancient beginnings of humankind, it is yet adaptable to the needs of modern society, basically because it involves simple human to human contact in an increasingly complex world. At first glance, shiatsu may be seen as only a series of techniques, and once a practitioner has learned a routine, that is sufficient. The strength of the shiatsu treatment, however, is the practitioner's knowledge base. The aim of this book is to provide that knowledge base and methods used in shiatsu. In other words, this book aims to bridge theory and technique.

The traditional Asian view of health and harmony (traditional Chinese medicine) is the foundation on which the techniques are built, and this book presents the information in easy to digest sections. Traditional Chinese medicine does not need to seem mysterious or difficult. Instead, it can be thought of as a natural outgrowth of human interaction with the Earth. Once practitioners understand this, they can interact with and educate their clients on a deeper level. This, in turn, can lead to greater awareness of shiatsu, on a local, regional, and national level.

WHO WILL BENEFIT FROM THIS BOOK?

The Practice of Shiatsu grew out of a need for a concise, comprehensive textbook and workbook that can be used for many shiatsu programs. It is designed as a teaching aid for entry-level shiatsu students or students who have had a small amount of shiatsu training. Massage therapists or other bodyworkers who are learning shiatsu, either as a continuing education course or within a primary massage therapy program, can also benefit from using *The Practice of Shiatsu.*

The book can be adapted to courses of varying lengths and depth and encompasses all the elements necessary to teach students to become successful shiatsu practitioners. The approach is to teach complex Eastern philosophies, theories, and ideas in ways that are understandable to students in Western culture. Foundational information and techniques are taught first; then more complex material is introduced to allow students time to integrate the material. Simple techniques are shown first, and as students master these, additional techniques designed for skill enhancement are presented. Good body mechanics is emphasized throughout. All of this will serve students well in their bodywork practice, preventing injury and ensuring longevity in the profession.

ORGANIZATION

Although shiatsu in and of itself is a fairly recent modality, its roots are deep. Along with the evolution of shiatsu, how traditional Chinese medicine and ancient Asian healing techniques provide the framework for the development of shiatsu is discussed in the first section of this book. Included in this discussion are Qi (Ki) and Qi connection, Yin and Yang, Vital Substances, Five Element Theory, causes of disease according to traditional Chinese medicine, organs, channels (meridians), tsubo, hara, kyo, jitsu, and the Four Methods of Assessments. Also included is a section on Qigong to assist students in cultivating their own Qi and to develop their ability to connect with their clients' Qi.

Concluding the first section, a routine, called a *kata*, is outlined for students to follow to learn basic shiatsu techniques and body mechanics.

Throughout Section Two, information is presented for students to begin the process of integrating theory and practice by continuing to develop their touch sensitivity, outlining the components of the treatment session, conducting pretreatment interviews, and performing assessments. This is continued through emphasis on moving beyond the *kata* into determining imbalances in one or more of the Five Elements. Students learn to perform treatments that are more client centered and include specific work on one or more channels, as well as recommendations for client self-care.

For enhancement of the growth of students' shiatsu treatments in a personal, creative style, additional techniques are provided in the last chapter. These include ways to work the hara, anterior legs and arms, neck, face, back, posterior legs, and more side position techniques. Body mechanics are reinforced throughout all techniques.

DISTINCTIVE TEXTBOOK FEATURES AND PEDAGOGY

Because shiatsu is essentially learned by doing, it is important that students have relevant, readily applicable material to learn from. Distinctive features make this book both a textbook and a workbook and provide methods for students to learn visually, auditorily, and kinesthetically. These features include the following:

- Small blocks of text
- Color photos of all techniques

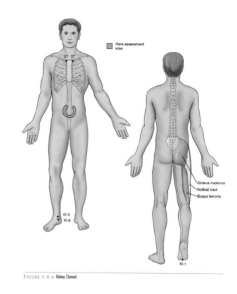

FIGURE 5-8 ■ Kidney Channel.

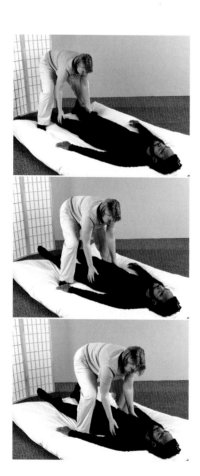

- Clear diagrams illustrating vital information, such as Five Element cycles and hara assessment
- Concrete examples of imbalances in each of the Five Elements and how to address them
- Margin notes of important and interesting information

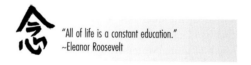

"All of life is a constant education."
~Eleanor Roosevelt

- Bibliography

In addition, there are learning aids for students:

- Key terms at the beginning of each chapter
- Learning objectives at the beginning of each chapter

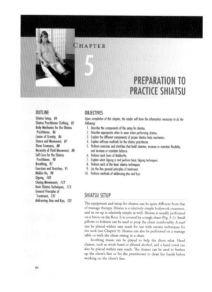

- Color diagrams of all channels (meridians) and commonly used points (tsubo)

- Glossary of terms
- Workbook activities that include the following:
  - Blank human figures on which students can draw each of the channels (meridians)
  - Fill-in questions
  - Suggested drawings to demonstrate concepts
  - How students should practice outside of class
  - How students should write up practice treatments outside of class
  - How to design a shiatsu intake form

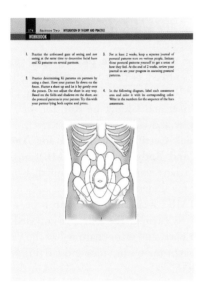

DVD

Available to students at the back of the book is a DVD with almost 2 hours of proper shiatsu techniques and a sample pretreatment interview. The book is supported by this DVD, which is playable both in set-top DVD players and in computers, and which includes video showing the specific applications and techniques described in the book. Each video clip on the DVD is referenced in the book through double-numbered icons directing the students to where they can find particular clips on the DVD.

Examples of video clips include the following:
- Exercise and stretches
- Basic shiatsu techniques
- Basic Kata, including the hara techniques
- A standard treatment session
- Examples of the Five Elements

NOTE TO THE STUDENT

Because *The Practice of Shiatsu* has both theory and technique, students should consider both of them equally when learning shiatsu. Theory can come alive when students are willing to think of and view the world in new ways, ask questions, and are open to changes in themselves. A natural result of this will be awareness of their own and their client's Qi, which in turn spurs growth as a shiatsu practitioner. Because the only way to get better at doing shiatsu is to practice shiatsu, students should make time for this important aspect of learning. The more the student practices, the more the theory becomes integrated and the more useful theory becomes. This continues to be true as the student becomes a professional and throughout the professional shiatsu practitioner's career. *The Practice of Shiatsu* should be used as a guide to this process. By serving as a foundation, it can be a useful reference for professionals as they become more expert.

Sandra K. Anderson
Tucson, Arizona
June 2007

ACKNOWLEDGMENTS

Sara Harders, who kindly agreed to be photographed as the other shiatsu practitioner in this book. Her innate sense of Qi and natural, fluid movements ensure her a long and fulfilling career as a professional bodyworker.

Bob Lehnberg, whose gentleness belies his strength and whose calm demeanor is a gateway to an inquisitive and insightful mind. He teaches by example.

Cora Jacobson, a devoted and disciplined fellow instructor. She created fun and innovative teaching methods.

Tama Hader, friend and fellow instructor, whose commitment and dedication to shiatsu always made me be sure that I brought my best into the classroom.

Terry Norman, a lifelong learner and teacher of Asian bodywork. He provided invaluable historical and technical information.

Michaela Johnson, for her careful scrutiny of this text and her ability to get right to the heart of the matter.

Heidi Wilson, for her embodiment of subtlety; she helped me develop the ability to feel energy on many different levels.

Kris Schaefer, whose teaching made me understand the grace of shiatsu.

Leslie McGee, an acupuncturist who made traditional Chinese medicine come alive and make sense. Her down-to-earth style and humor made her classes a joy.

Suzan Fleck, who taught me that shiatsu requires focus and specificity, as well as art and dance.

Yoshi Nakano, a master shiatsu practitioner and teacher. His wisdom, experience, and humor help me find my center.

Jan Schwartz, for her support of me as a teacher and a professional bodyworker.

Joann Rockwell MacMaster, a shiatsu receiver and friend who has helped me define what is proper and real.

Margaret Avery Moon, one of the founders of the Desert Institute of the Healing Arts, the setting in which I learned shiatsu and honed my teaching skills.

Kathy Rinn, for being a mentor and a friend. She showed me the way when I began my professional bodywork career.

All the models in the photographs and **DVD,** who gave so freely of their time and bodies!

Jeanne Robertson, for her outstanding artwork.

Jim Visser and **Chuck Le Roi,** for their excellent photography and videography, respectively.

National Certification Board for Therapeutic Massage and Bodywork (NCBTMB), an organization that I have volunteered for and that has helped me foster my leadership abilities.

NCBTMB's Examination Committee, a committee I formerly chaired. The collective knowledge, expertise, experience, and razor-sharp wit of the Committee members kept me on my toes and striving for correct information.

Garnet Adair, Carol Davis, and **Annie Gordon,** because they are true friends who have provided unlimited support, laughter, and common sense.

My animal companions throughout my life, because it has been through them that I had my first understanding of Qi and connection.

I have been a professional bodyworker and bodywork educator for 16 years. Because of my students, clients, fellow instructors, and fellow bodyworkers, every day has been a day of learning, opportunity, and growth. Without them, I never would have truly understood or been mindful of just how important and powerful human to human connection and caring touch are.

CONTENTS

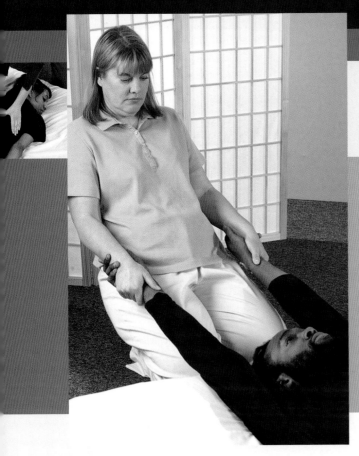

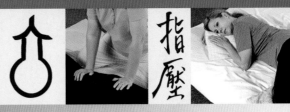

THE FUNDAMENTALS OF SHIATSU

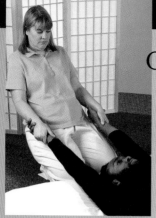

CHAPTER

1

HISTORY OF SHIATSU

OBJECTIVES

Upon completion of this chapter, the reader will have the information necessary to do the following:
1. Explain the differences between how a massage therapy treatment is performed and how a shiatsu treatment is performed.
2. Describe the Western view of disease versus the Eastern view of disharmony in the human body.
3. Explain the similarities and differences shiatsu has to acupuncture.
4. Describe the indications and contraindications for shiatsu.
5. Briefly trace the development of An Wu to Anma to shiatsu.
6. Explain Namikoshi's influence in the practice of shiatsu.
7. Explain Masunaga's influence in the practice of shiatsu.
8. Describe the different types of shiatsu.

S hiatsu is a wonderful and unique type of bodywork. It was born of the human need to touch others and to make others feel better by being touched. It grew out of the ancient connection of human beings to the earth, to the universe, and to each other. It combines art and science, theory and practice, strength and softness, intellect and intuition. It is about supporting and it is about letting go, and knowing when to do which. **Shiatsu** can be performed as a dance, and like any dance done well, many hours of study and practice go into making it look and feel effortless.

"True art takes note not merely of form but also of what lies behind."
~Mahatma Gandhi

Key Terms

Shiatsu is a relatively young bodywork practice. Its roots, however, extend deep into millennia of **traditional Chinese medicine**. Its techniques come from systems developed by common folk, imperial physicians, blind practitioners, and physicians for the samurai. Having learned these historical techniques, contemporary practitioners also contribute their own unique methods and ideas. The beauty of shiatsu is its ability to retain foundational principles and evolve at the same time. Although it is of the past, it is also a living bodywork form that adapts, changes, and grows.

WHAT IS SHIATSU?

Although it does have some elements in common with Western massage therapy and many other types of bodywork, shiatsu should not be mistaken for massage. Occasionally the term "shiatsu massage" is used, which is in reality a combination of two different types of bodywork. To be accurate, "shiatsu" and "massage" should be thought of as separate terms.

Western massage therapy is based on Western views of the body—namely the scientific study of anatomy, physiology, and kinesiology. The massage practitioner assesses the client's physical needs by observing, listening to the client, palpating soft tissue, and performing active and passive stretches with the client. Massage therapy typically is performed on a massage table, with the client unclothed and draped by sheets (Fig. 1-1).

A lubricant, such as oil or lotion, is applied to the client's skin. After warm-up techniques are performed, physical manipulation of the client's soft tissue is done to increase blood flow into tissues, release muscle tension, and elongate the fascia around muscles. Stretches and range of motion movements can be incorporated to lengthen muscle tissue and increase nutrition within the joints. The massage practitioner can use his or her hands, fingers, thumbs, forearms, and elbows to achieve the desired results of treatment. The massage practitioner's strength comes up from the legs and is transmitted through the shoulders and then out through the arms (Fig. 1-2).

Modern shiatsu includes knowledge of Western sciences but has a foundation in ancient Asian medicine; certain types of shiatsu also incorporate Asian philosophies. The basis of shiatsu is the concept that the client's "energy," which can be thought of as vitality or vigor, is out of balance in some way, resulting in pain, discomfort, or other disorders. The goal of shiatsu is to help rebalance the client's energy and alleviate discomfort. To assess the client's needs, the shiatsu practitioner observes, listens, palpates the client, and uses intuition. Shiatsu typically is performed on a futon (mat) on the floor, with the client wearing comfortable, loose-fitting clothes. No lubricants are used (Fig. 1-3). The shiatsu practitioner uses palpation, physical manipulation techniques, stretches, and range of motion movements to equilibriate the client's energy and to assist in moving it more evenly throughout the client's body. The shiatsu practitioner can use pressure from his or her palms, fingers, thumbs, forearms, elbows, knees, and feet during the course of the treatment. The shiatsu practitioner's strength comes from the center of his or her body (belly

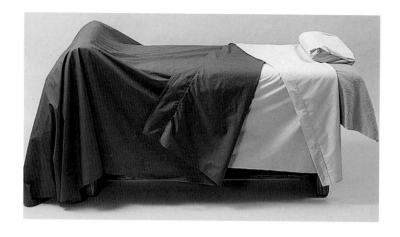

FIGURE 1-1 ■ Massage therapy set-up. (From Fritz S: *Mosby's fundamentals of therapeutic massage,* ed 3, St Louis, 2004, Mosby.)

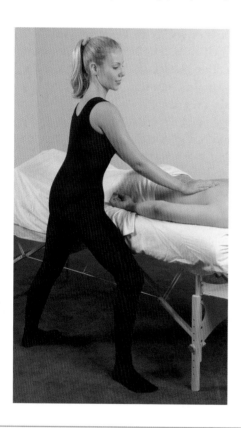

FIGURE 1-2 ■ Massage therapist performing a treatment. (From Salvo S: *Massage therapy: principles and practice,* ed. 3, St Louis, 2007, Saunders.)

and hips) and is transmitted outward through the extremities (Fig. 1-4).

Shiatsu is a Japanese form of bodywork, and as such embodies and reflects the culture of Japan.

It is firmly rooted in tradition yet is constantly melding and reinventing as new ideas, methods, and viewpoints are encountered. The ability to be both flexible and unyielding has enabled Japan to survive and flourish for thousands of years. This uniqueness of Japan is the same uniqueness of shiatsu.

Like all bodywork therapies, shiatsu has a rich and interesting history. As in all bodywork therapies, it developed from an accumulation of knowledge, experience, expertise, and trial and error. The result is an interesting compilation of principles that may seem to contradict each other. However, as in the general culture of Japan, the dichotomies of shiatsu are its strengths. They provide the framework for the flexibility necessary to perform shiatsu successfully.

The seeming contradictions of shiatsu can be seen even in its definition. In Japanese, *shi* means finger and *atsu* means pressure, so shiatsu is literally "finger pressure." However, this definition is overly simplistic. The implication is that all a practitioner needs to do to perform shiatsu is press her fingers onto another person's body, which is not the case.

Shiatsu treatment involves physicality (practitioners use their thumbs, fingers, palms, forearms, elbows, knees, and feet), but practitioners use their intuition as well (Fig. 1-5). In fact, the physical movements practitioners use are guided by their perceptions and insight gained through trusting their intuition.

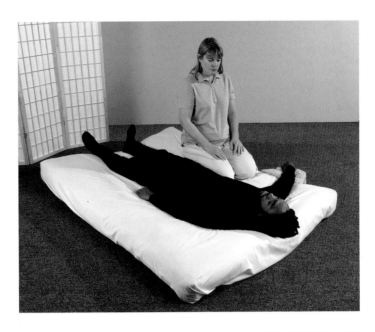

FIGURE 1-3 ▪ Shiatsu set-up.

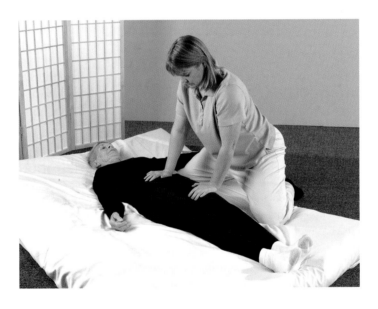

FIGURE 1-4 ▪ Shiatsu practitioner performing a treatment.

WESTERN ANATOMY AND PHYSIOLOGY AND TRADITIONAL CHINESE MEDICINE

Knowledge of Western anatomy and physiology, as well as knowledge of traditional Chinese medicine, provides the practitioner with additional expertise to draw from. Western science and traditional Chinese medicine are somewhat themselves contradictory components of shiatsu. Western anatomy and physiology deal with the physical structure of the body. With the belief that to understand the whole one must understand the parts, the study of the body starts with its cells and works up to tissues, organs, and systems. Disorders and diseases are characterized by signs and symptoms. Western treatment of diseases and

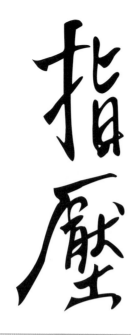

FIGURE 1-5 ■ Kanji for "shiatsu." **Kanji** is the Japanese writing system that uses characters adapted from Chinese.

disorders involves pinpointing the cause and then eliminating or alleviating it.

The shiatsu practitioner should have knowledge of Western anatomy and physiology to understand the physical structure and functioning of the human body. In addition, this text is written for practitioners of shiatsu in Western culture, whose clients will have experienced only Western medicine. A common view of the human body can provide a starting point for shiatsu practitioners to educate their clients about the Eastern philosophical view of the body, or traditional Chinese medicine.

Traditional Chinese medicine views the entire human being as body, mind, and spirit. Every living thing is part of the greater continuum of its environment, the Earth, and the universe. **Qi** (pronounced "chee") is the energy or force that gives and maintains life (the body's "energy," discussed previously) and also is the connection between organisms and all creation. Optimally, Qi flows within living creatures in a balanced, harmonious way, sustaining health. If Qi is not flowing properly, disharmony and lack of balance result, resulting in illness. Many treatments to restore the harmonious balance of Qi are based on traditional Chinese medicine. Some examples are **herbal therapy**, **moxibustion** (applying herbal

heat to specific points on the body), **acupuncture** and, of course, shiatsu.

Shiatsu is based on the same principles as is acupuncture. These include the concept that Qi (Ki in Japanese) flows in specific streams in the body called **channels**, or **meridians**. These channels are connected to the organs of the body and share the name of the organ. Examples are the Lung Channel, Large Intestine Channel, Stomach Channel, and Spleen Channel. The organs and channels have certain physical, mental, psychological, emotional, and spiritual functions in the body, and the balanced flow of Qi in the channels sustains these functions. This is discussed in further detail in Chapter 3.

Along the channels are points where the Qi is accessed easily. When the flow of Qi is disrupted for any of many possible reasons, it can be brought back into equilibrium by affecting the Qi at the points. Acupuncturists insert needles into the points to balance Qi. Shiatsu practitioners, however, use their own Qi to support and stabilize their client's Qi. They do this through physical manipulation—finger pressure, thumb pressure, palming, stretches, and range of motion. Some types of shiatsu mainly focus on addressing points; other types address the entire channel (Fig. 1-6).

WHO CAN RECEIVE SHIATSU?

Shiatsu can be appealing to many different persons. It can be performed on the old and the young, those in excellent health and those in fragile health, those who are experienced in receiving many different types of bodywork and those who have never received any type of bodywork at all. It may be especially attractive to those who feel uncomfortable removing their clothes for a massage treatment.

People can receive shiatsu for relaxation or to help them with specific conditions. In particular, shiatsu can help alleviate insomnia, anxiety, depression, headaches, muscular tension, digestive tract issues, and sinus congestion. In some cases it can also help increase local circulation and the movement of lymph.

Sometimes conditions that are contraindicated for massage therapy are not contraindicated for shiatsu. For example, the flare-up stages of

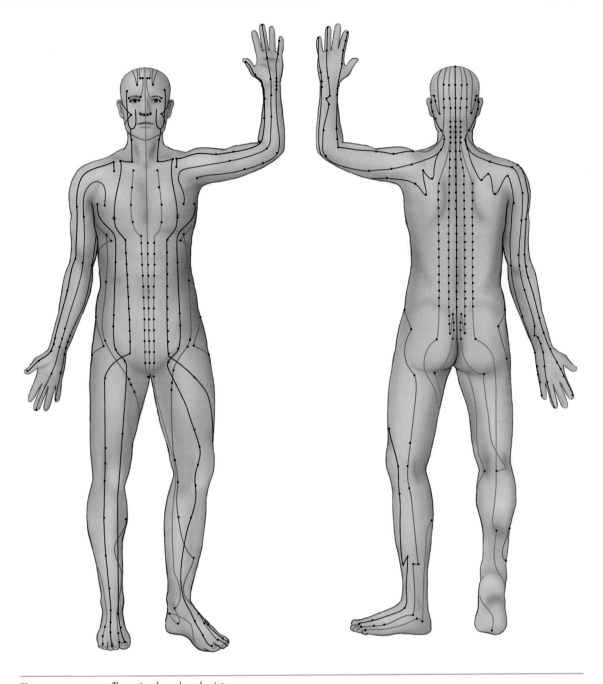

FIGURE 1-6 ▪ The major channels and points.

autoimmune diseases such as lupus and rheumatoid arthritis are contraindications for massage therapy because massage techniques can stimulate the production of histamine, which would further exacerbate the inflammation that occurs during the flare-up stage. Also, the massage techniques may simply be too painful for the person to receive. Instead, shiatsu could be performed with clearance from the client's health care provider. Stretches and range of motion techniques would be contraindicated. However, the simple act of the shiatsu practitioner placing his or her hands on the client and making a Qi connection may help the client feel better. If the client cannot tolerate touch, shiatsu can be performed energetically above the person.

Certain conditions warrant caution for the practice of shiatsu. For clients who have debilitating conditions such as osteoporosis, or those undergoing chemotherapy, only the lightest pressure or energetic work above the body should be performed. The application of shiatsu techniques also has local contraindications such as varicose veins, wounds, bone fractures, recent scars, and areas of inflammation. Inflamed, painful joints, including arthritic joints, are contraindications for range of motion techniques. Also, any vertebral column issues, such as a herniated disc or ankylosing spondylitis, are contraindications for certain range of motion techniques and across-the-body stretches. These are further described in subsequent chapters discussing specific shiatsu techniques.

DEVELOPMENT OF ASIAN BODYWORK

Stone needles have been found in Neolithic (or New Stone Age) sites in China that date as far back as 8000 BC. These implements were thought to be used to stimulate points and channels. Because touch is the most instinctive form of comfort and healing, points and channels likely were pressed and massaged with fingers and palms long before needles were used. The origins of shiatsu, and all forms of bodywork, then predate the use of tools. Bodywork could be said to have begun the first time one human being reached out to touch another human being with good intention.

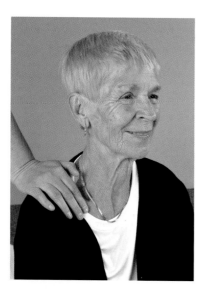

EARLY CHINESE BODYWORK

Over time, the natural instinct to touch one another gradually developed into the earliest forms of bodywork. Because this was before recorded history, how touching and pressing became systemized into modalities is unknown. What is known is that the oldest forms of treatment in Asia, **An Wu** and Do-In, developed in China more than 5000 years ago.

An Wu resembled Western massage. It consisted of pressing, gliding, stretching, and percussing the body. The practitioner used his or her thumbs, fingers, forearms, elbows, knees, and feet on the points along the channels of Qi flow. **Do-In** (or **Tao-Yinn**) was similar to yoga. It is still being practiced today as a combination of exercises for channel stretching, breathing, Qi flow, and self-massage.

At the same time that these early forms of bodywork were being formalized, traditional Chinese medicine precepts were being developed. In brief, the ancient Chinese viewed themselves as part of nature and the universe around them, with Qi as a unifying factor. Because their view of health and disease was that both are on a continuum of Qi flow, An Wu, Do-In, and traditional Chinese medicine naturally developed together. (More will be discussed about this in Chapter 2.) As ancient practitioners worked with Chinese medicine and physical manipulation techniques on the body, they became their culture's physicians. The healing properties of plants were studied and incorporated into treatments; this became Chinese herbal medicine. Shen Nung, one of the first five emperors, dating back before 2700 BC, is credited with creating herbal medicine in China.

Gradually, An Wu came to be known as Anmo, which began to become popular as a medical treatment. By the fifth century, Anmo had developed into a more sophisticated system of theory, diagnosis, and treatment and was being studied as a doctoral degree in the State Office of Imperial Physicians. During this time Anmo spread to other Asian countries such as Korea, Japan, and India. By the 1300s, however, Anmo had become less popular and was being used less as a medical procedure. Better Anmo techniques continued to be developed, though, such as procedures to ease childbirth. Anmo especially focused on musculoskeletal disorders and injuries, which laid the foundations for the practice of medical bone setting called **Tuina**.

During the Ming Dynasty (1368-1644), a resurgence in Anmo occurred. Imperial physicians again considered Anmo a viable medical treatment, although the term Tuina began to be used in place of Anmo. This marked a division in views of bodywork. Anmo continued to be practiced, but Tuina was considered more "scientific." Today in China Anmo is referred to as "folk massage" and is practiced more for relaxation and stress relief, whereas Tuina is referred as "medical massage" and is performed in hospitals and clinics.

Throughout the ages, as more and more physicians palpated and massaged patients, they pinpointed the effects of pressing certain locations on Qi channels. They also discovered that more specific pressure on these more specific locations had greater effect. These locations on Qi channels were narrowed down into points. Over time, pressure on these points became more and more precise, until needles were finally inserted into the points, giving birth to acupuncture. The points were named, numbered, and classified in the system that is still used today. This system is common to both acupuncture and shiatsu.

Acupuncture gradually took over in China as the primary form of medicine. However, palpatory and massage (Anmo, Tuina, and Do-In) techniques remained important foundational techniques. Physicians had to master bodywork before they were allowed to progress to using needles. Even though acupuncture became the primary form of healing, massaging (as in rubbing and pressing the channels and points) remained quite popular.

The theory of Qi and traditional Chinese medicine traveled throughout Asia, and so did hands-on physical manipulation. Tibet, the Philippines, Indonesia, and Thailand all have their own traditional medicine and bodywork modalities that have at least some elements in common with traditional Chinese medicine and Anmo.

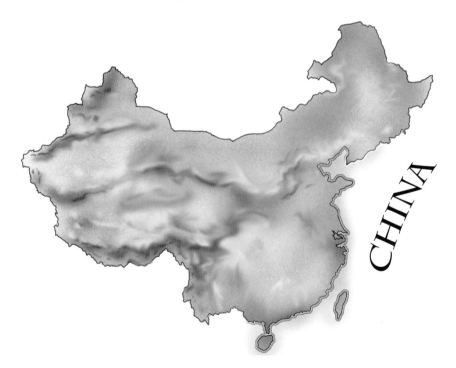

CHINA

FROM CHINA TO JAPAN

Because of geographic proximity, Japanese culture and Chinese culture have had a close relationship. During the sixth century AD, monks from China traveling to Japan brought combinations of Chinese philosophies that included Buddhism, Taoism, and Confucianism. They also brought knowledge of Chinese medicine. Trading between China and Japan opened up more communication between the two countries, and Japanese students were sent to China to learn more about Chinese culture and medicine.

Acupuncture and Anmo, with their basis on Qi, were readily infused into Japanese culture. As the years progressed, acupuncture remained relatively the same as when it arrived in Japan. However, Anmo was modified and refined to fit Japanese culture and gradually evolved into **Anma**, or **Amma**. Japan's early history was marked by many warring states and no unified central government. By 1185, these states were known as shogunates, and their leaders were called shoguns. They had highly trained, armed men called samurai to fight their battles. The fighting techniques the samurai used are the origins of modern Japanese martial arts. The medical practitioners in Japan were expected to keep these men healthy and fit. Anma became a mixture of the original Anmo techniques imported from China and techniques specifically developed for samurai needs.

During the Edo period (1602-1868) Anma reached its height of popularity. New Anma techniques and methods were developed, schools were established, and texts were written to teach Anma. The shogunates had been organized into a functioning country ruled by one shogun appointed by Japan's emperor. Along the way, the samurai lost most of their importance. Over time, their fighting techniques meshed more with Buddhist, Tao, and Confucian philosophies than with actual combat, and the modern martial arts were born.

Also during this time, Japan was closed to the west. Shogun Ieyasu, the country's principal leader, viewed European culture as a threat to the new national stability and instigated a closed-door policy. This policy prevented all cultural and political contact with the outside world. The Dutch were the only people allowed to trade with Japan, and contact was limited to a small island off Nagasaki. The Dutch introduced Western medical information, including anatomy and physiology, to the Japanese; the Japanese taught Anma and acupuncture to the Dutch, who took these modalities back to Europe.

Not many professions were open to the visually impaired during this period. Anma was available to them, however, with the reasoning that the blind have greater touch sensitivity. It was also seen as a form of welfare. Soon Anma was being practiced mostly by blind practitioners, and because being visually impaired limited the education these practitioners were able to receive throughout this period, their medical knowledge fell below that of the physicians and herbalists. Much technical and clinical wisdom was lost, and Anma became known as being useful only for relaxation.

WESTERN INFLUENCE

In 1854 American Naval Commodore Matthew C. Perry virtually forced Japan to open to trade with the Western world. In 1853, he had ported ships near Edo (today known as Tokyo) and was met by representatives of the Tokugawa shogunate. They told Perry to proceed to Nagasaki, the only Japanese port open to foreigners at that time. Perry refused to leave and demanded permission to present a letter from President Millard Fillmore

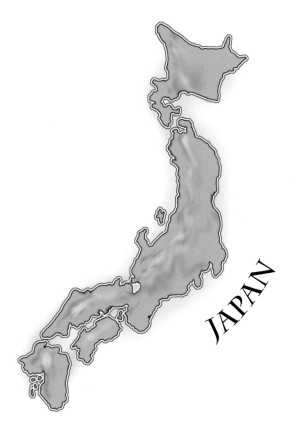

allowing trade between Japan and the United States. He threatened force if he was denied. The Japanese military could not withstand Perry's weaponry, so they let him come ashore to avoid being bombarded. Perry presented President Fillmore's letter and left for China, promising to return for a reply. Perry returned to Japan in 1854 with twice as many ships. A treaty fulfilling all the demands in Fillmore's letter had been prepared. Perry signed the treaty, called the Convention of Kanagawa, on March 31, 1854, and departed.

This agreement helped lead to the fall of shoguns and the ascent of imperialism. The Meiji period of Japan (1868-1912) saw an overhaul of the Japanese government. It was re-created in a Western framework, and changes were instigated to make Japanese society more like Western society. Western medicine dominated, and traditional medicine was relegated to the realm of folk medicine. The therapeutic value of Anma and Asian medicine was rejected, although segments of the population still retained their attachment to these practices and Anma remained an occupation for the blind. Also during this time Western massage therapy was introduced to Japan.

By the beginning of the 1900s, Anma had lost so much credibility that it was considered shady employment. The practitioners of the true art of Anma sought a way to distinguish themselves from charlatans and "body shampooers." A new name was needed, and in 1919, Tamai Tempaku published a book called *Shiatsu Ho,* which translates to "finger pressure method." This text united Anma and Western anatomy and physiology and used concepts from **Ampuku** (abdominal massage) and Do-In.

Shiatsu began to develop a different look from the established techniques and principles used in authentic Anma. The Japanese ability to be flexible while still honoring tradition is exemplified by the path shiatsu has taken. Shiatsu practitioners started merging Western bodywork techniques from chiropractic medicine and massage therapy with conventional Anma methods. Western medicine concepts such as anatomy, physiology, and psychology were used along with traditional Chinese medicine theory.

In 1925 the Shiatsu Therapists' Association was formed to promote shiatsu as a legitimate profession and to distinguish it from Anma. Also in 1925 Tokujiro Namikoshi (1905-2000) founded the Clinic of Pressure Therapy in Hokkaido, Japan. As a child, Namikoshi discovered his gift for manual therapy by helping alleviate his mother's rheumatoid arthritis symptoms. He went on to study Anma and Western massage therapy. Because he studied both subjects, his focus was to practice shiatsu within a Western structure. He did not emphasize the study of channels. Instead, he concentrated on knowledge of the physical structure of the body and the nervous system and stressed the anatomic locations of points. The Namikoshi style of shiatsu involves applying methodical patterns of pressure along the points.

NAMIKOSHI

In the successive years, both the conventional and Western (Namikoshi) styles of shiatsu were taught and practiced. In 1933, Namikoshi went to Tokyo to teach shiatsu. In 1940 he opened the Japan Shiatsu Institute, which helped further awareness of shiatsu as a valid profession. However, after the defeat of Japan in World War II, aspects of traditional Japanese culture were suppressed. In this atmosphere and spirit General Douglas MacArthur prohibited the practice of shiatsu and Anma. The practitioners of these modalities were forced underground. Because many Anma practitioners and many shiatsu practitioners were blind, this prohibition denied them a way of making a living. Helen Keller intervened on their behalf and the ban was lifted (Fig. 1-7).

In 1955 the Japanese government officially recognized shiatsu as a part of Anma. This was the

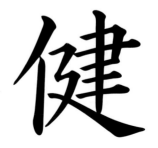

FIGURE 1-7 ■ Kanji for "health."

first legal sanction of shiatsu. In 1957 Namikoshi's Japan Shiatsu Institute was officially licensed as the Japan Shiatsu School by the Minister of Health and Welfare. The school proved to be enormously popular, and Namikoshi's son, Toru, went on to teach shiatsu in Europe and the United States, thus helping spread shiatsu beyond Japan's borders.

MASUNAGA

Shizuto Masunaga (1925-1981) was born into a family of shiatsu practitioners. His mother had studied with Tamai Tempaku, the author of *Shiatsu Ho*. Because of his mother's influence, Masunaga was quite interested in traditional Asian medicine. Although he chose to study Western psychology, he also studied ancient Chinese medical texts and maintained an interest in Asian spiritual philosophies. After studying psychology, Masunaga decided to pursue his interest in shiatsu. He attended Namikoshi's Japan Shiatsu School and then taught there for 10 years. He was also a professor of psychology at Tokyo University while he taught psychology at the Japan Shiatsu School.

In a natural progression, Masunaga began blending his areas of expertise. He integrated conventional shiatsu, ancient Asian medicine, psychology, and Western physiology. His approach focused more on assessing the body's Qi patterns and, instead of simply targeting specific points, concentrated on addressing appropriate channels to adjust and rebalance Qi flow. Masunaga also introduce the concepts of support and connection by the shiatsu practitioner by using both hands, a sustaining "mother hand" and a working "son hand." He incorporated aspects of spirituality used by Zen Buddhist monks.

He also discovered, through palpation and personal insight, the existence in the body of extensions of the classic channels. For example, certain classic channels are found only in the arms. Masunaga discovered that extensions of these channels are also found in the legs. Certain other classic channels are found only in the legs; Masunaga delineated extensions of these channels in the arms.

These extensions mean that nearly every channel can be addressed in every area of the body. Masunaga called this new style **Zen shiatsu**. He opened the Iokai Shiatsu Center in Tokyo to teach his style of shiatsu. The development of Zen shiatsu typifies the history of shiatsu—a mixture of ancient and modern, Eastern and Western, science and intuition.

TYPES OF SHIATSU

Because shiatsu is a mixture of traditional and modern concepts and techniques, evolution is inherent in this type of bodywork. The nature of shiatsu is innovation. Many modern derivatives exist; each combines components of the two major types of shiatsu, Namikoshi's style and Masunaga's style. Following is a brief explanation of the most common types of shiatsu currently practiced. All styles of shiatsu entail manipulation of Qi in some way to affect harmony in the client's body.

NAMIKOSHI SHIATSU

As previously discussed, **Namikoshi shiatsu**, also called **Nippon shiatsu**, was developed by Namikoshi and is quite common in Japan. It involves a whole-body routine that incorporates stretches, but the emphasis is more on points than channels. It tends to be a vigorous treatment.

TSUBO THERAPY AND ACUPRESSURE

The Japanese word for a **point** on a channel is **tsubo**. Katsusuke Serizawa, a contemporary of Namikoshi and Masunaga, concentrated on tsubo. He proved their existence scientifically by measuring their electrical activity on the skin. He emphasized stimulating tsubo, whether through moxibustion, acupuncture, or finger pressure. **Acupressure** is the Western derivative of **tsubo therapy**, which involves working the tsubo by pressing with the fingers.

ZEN SHIATSU

As previously discussed, Zen shiatsu was developed by Masunaga and also is popular in Japan. Treatment emphasis is more on the channels than the tsubo. The practitioner's intuition and connection with the client's Qi is vital. The treatment can be either gentle or vigorous.

OHASHIATSU

Ohashiatsu was developed by Wataru Ohashi, who opened the Shiatsu Institute in New York City in 1974. Ohashiatsu focuses less on finger pressure along the channels and more on stretching and physically manipulating the client's body to achieve Qi balance.

FIVE ELEMENT SHIATSU

Five Element shiatsu focuses on patterns of disharmony in the Five Element Cycle (defined in Chapter 2) as an assessment tool. The treatment plan uses techniques to balance the client's Qi and restore the harmony of the Five Element Cycle.

MACROBIOTIC SHIATSU

Macrobiotic, or **barefoot**, **shiatsu** was developed by Shizuko Yamamoto and combines macrobiotic nutritional principles with shiatsu techniques to assist clients in their health and healing processes. This style of shiatsu combines pressure on tsubo with stretches and physical manipulation. It is also called barefoot shiatsu because practitioners originally used their bare feet to apply many techniques. Currently barefoot shiatsu means techniques specifically applied with the feet, whether they are bare or have socks on them.

Of note, this text does not promote one style of shiatsu over another and instead incorporates aspects of many different styles.

WORKBOOK

1. Differentiate between the components of a massage therapy treatment and the components of a shiatsu treatment by listing them below in their respective columns.

	Massage Therapy	Shiatsu
Basis	_____	_____
Equipment	_____	_____
	_____	_____
	_____	_____
Source of practitioner's strength	_____	_____
Parts of practitioner's body used	_____	_____
	_____	_____

2. List three conditions that could benefit from shiatsu and three conditions that are contraindications for shiatsu.

Benefit from Shiatsu	Contraindications for Shiatsu
_____	_____
_____	_____
_____	_____

3. Draw a timeline showing the events in the development of shiatsu.

4.   List the characteristics of each type of shiatsu.

Type of Shiatsu	Characteristics
Namikoshi	_____
	_____
	_____
Tsubo therapy/	_____
acupressure	_____
	_____
Zen shiatsu	_____
	_____
	_____
Ohashiatsu	_____
	_____
	_____
Five Element shiatsu	_____
	_____
	_____
Macrobiotic (barefoot)	_____
shiatsu	_____
	_____

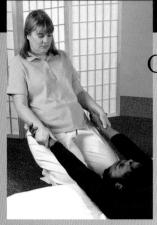

CHAPTER

2

FOUNDATIONS OF ASIAN MEDICINE

OBJECTIVES

Upon completion of this chapter, the reader will have the information necessary to do the following:
1. Explain the importance of learning Western anatomy, physiology, and pathology as well as traditional Chinese medicine for shiatsu.
2. Briefly describe the development of traditional Chinese medicine up to and including *The Yellow Emperor's Classic of Internal Medicine.*
3. Explain the concepts and interrelations of Yin and Yang.
4. List examples of Yin and Yang phenomena.
5. List examples of Yin and Yang in the human body.
6. Explain what Qi is and where it comes from.
7. Describe Qi's roles in the human body.
8. Describe each of the Vital Substances.
9. Describe each of the causes of disease according to traditional Chinese medicine.

Shiatsu techniques can be learned, and protocols can be followed. The same treatment can be given over and over without much thought given to the theoretic basis of Asian bodywork. However, doing the same routine by rote, or with minimal variety, serves neither clients nor the practitioner well. The most effective and interesting treatments are those born of harmony between practice and theory.

Practice involves learning techniques and proper mechanics. By learning from a skilled instructor, the shiatsu practitioner acquires a variety of techniques for any area of the client's body and any of a variety of disorders the client may be experiencing. Practice also means honing skills through consistently working on a range of clients—different ages, levels of vitality, body shapes and sizes, and so on. Over time, applying shiatsu methods to many clients develops a practitioner's awareness, connection, and intuition, which are crucial to the

Bad Diet
Blood
Body Fluids
Cold
Constitution
Damp
Damp-Cold
Damp-Heat
Dryness
Excess Sexual Activity
External Causes of Disease
Heat

Huang Ti Nei Ching (The
    Yellow Emperor's Classic of
    Internal Medicine)
Incorrect Treatment
Internal Causes of Disease
Internal Cold
Internal Dampness
Internal Dryness
Internal Heat
Internal Wind
Jing
Kidney Essence

Organs
Overexertion
Parasites
Pernicious Influences
Poisons
Postnatal (Acquired) Essence
Prenatal (Congenital) Essence
Qi
Shen
Source Qi
Summer Heat

Tao
Trauma
Underexertion
Vital Substances
Weak Constitution
Wei Qi
Wind
Wind-Cold
Wind-Damp
Wind-Heat
Yin and Yang

work of shiatsu. Without these, performing shiatsu becomes a series of procedures done to the client, not the therapeutic experience that culminates when practitioner and client work in concert.

The cultivation of intuition, connection, and awareness, however, is accomplished only partially through practice. The other necessary component is knowledge gained from the study of Western anatomy, physiology, and pathology; Asian bodywork assessment techniques; and traditional Chinese medicine. All these subjects give the shiatsu practitioner more information to draw from, more tools to use, and a wider range of experience to build on. Many pieces of data form the mosaic of intuitive insight, and the practitioner should be open to as many sources of these data as possible.

Traditional Chinese medicine forms the foundation of Asian bodywork. When looked at from a Western viewpoint, traditional Chinese medicine may seem complicated and steeped in folklore. Placing Eastern medicine within a Western framework, though, can lead to confusion and skepticism, which are often seen when a person from Western culture initially studies Eastern bodywork. If, however, traditional Chinese medicine is considered as a body of knowledge within its own right, its theory, principles, and teachings make sense and can be used to enhance the personal development of both practitioner and client.

DEVELOPMENT OF TRADITIONAL CHINESE MEDICINE

The ancient Chinese were an agricultural people. They lived on and of the earth. Their very survival depended on understanding and living with the cycles of the weather, the seasons, and the sun and the moon. One season flows into the next, the moon waxes and wanes, clouds build into a summer storm, rain falls, and blue sky reappears. Over thousands of years the people understood the universe, the earth, nature, and themselves as all interconnected. Every living creature's life cycle is a microcosm of a large cycle involving the heavens and the earth. **Qi** is the life force or energy driving and connecting these cycles. Traditional Chinese medicine has its origins in these natural processes.

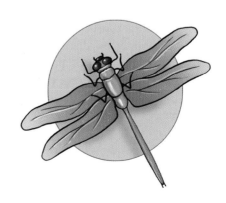

Chinese medicine developed in a region-specific manner. In other words, certain practices were cultivated according to the needs of the people in those regions. In northern China, moxibustion was used to counteract the lung issues the cold climate caused. In the south, the climate is warm and humid and the people tended to develop muscle cramps and muscles spasms. Pressing points alleviated them. First the fingers were used to press, then sharp stones, then needles, until acupuncture became the treatment of choice in the south. In western China, the land is mountainous and forested, and there are many different native plants. The use of medicinal herbs became predominant. In the rest of China, massage (first called Anwu, then called Anmo) became the treatment of choice.

Around 2700 BC, by order of the Chinese emporer, all the regional medical practices were studied and tested to see which ones were effective and practicable. This intense medical research yielded new techniques in both acupuncture and massage. Texts were written that detailed causes of disease and disorders and their Chinese medicinal treatments. These texts are thought to be the basis of the **Huang Ti Nei Ching (The Yellow Emperor's Classic of Internal Medicine)**, which was written much later.

During the end of the Qin Dynasty (221-206 BC) and throughout the Han Dynasty (206 BC-220 AD), education became more important in China. The *Book of the Mountains and the Seas* was written and included study of geography, natural philosophy, the animal and plant world, and popular myths. Sima Qian, perhaps China's greatest historian, wrote *Records of the Historian,* or *Shiji,* which was one of China's first attempts to record history in an organized form. An important text written during this time that promoted a new way at looking at disease and illness was the *Shan Hun Lun,* written by Zhang Zhong Jing. Considered one of the most insightful books of Chinese medical history, *Shan Hun Lun* discussed illnesses and disorders caused by invasion of "cold" and "cold damage" to the body and Qi. During this time of enlightenment *The Yellow Emperor's Classic of Internal Medicine* was written.

The *Yellow Emperor's Classic of Internal Medicine* is a series of texts that contain the fundamentals of all branches of Chinese medicine. Chinese physicians today still practice the theories explained in this book. It was written in the form of a dialogue in which the emperor seeks information from his minister, Ch'I-Po, on all questions relating to health and the art of healing. Because of *The Yellow Emperor's Classic of Internal Medicine,* a structured educational system in traditional Chinese medicine was created under the auspices of the Emperor Huangdi. This system included school and texts devoted to acupuncture, herbal medicine, sexual practices, and curative exercises such as Do-In and Anmo. The Han Dynasty nurtured traditional Chinese medicine and allowed it to grow and expand into what it is today.

YIN AND YANG

Lao Tzu, who lived in the sixth century BC, wrote about the **Tao** in a book entitled the *Tao Te Ching. Tao* has been translated to mean "road, path, way, means, doctrine, "God," "the universe," "nature," and "that which is." Most refer to the Tao as meaning "the way" or "the path." In the text, he describes how everything in the universe formed from the "great ultimate source." Outside of this was only emptiness. The Tao is the primary law of the universe, the law that is the genesis for all other laws and principles of the workings of the universe and the world. In a real sense, the Tao cannot be known, understood, or defined. From this concept arose the two prime principles of **Yin and Yang**. The Tao is manifested through the actions and interactions of Yin and Yang, through which all of creation is arrayed. When Yin and Yang came together, Qi was released. The Qi created the Five Elements (see Chapter 3), and from the Five Elements everything else was created.

Yin and Yang are represented by a classic symbol (Fig. 2-1). They are pivotal to the traditional philosophy, science, and culture in China and Japan and are essential to understanding traditional Chinese medicine. To truly understand Yin and Yang, two apparently opposing thoughts must be held at the same time: in lightness there is dark, and in darkness there is light. In the Yin Yang symbol, the dark area has a seed of light, and the light area has a seed of dark. These seeds visually represent that many times descriptions and definitions depend on what the concept or thing being described is not. Light is not darkness; high is not low; complex is not simple.

The light and dark areas in the Yin Yang symbol are not static; one flows into the other. The concepts of Yin and Yang are not fixed; they are in constant movement, always transforming each other. They are the natural limits for each other; Yin can only go so far before it becomes Yang; Yang can only go so far before it becomes Yin. The coldness and darkness of winter (Yin) only last for so long until the warmth and light of spring (Yang) (Fig. 2-2). So Yin and Yang should not be thought of as absolutes, such as everything dark is Yin and everything light is Yang. Instead, there is a continuum, a relationship. For instance, morning hours are Yang, and afternoon hours are Yin. However, 11 AM is more Yin than 1 AM, and 11 PM is more Yang than 1 PM. The best example, however, involves the Earth's water cycle.

As the sun heats the Earth, water from the oceans, lakes, rivers, and streams evaporates (Yang process), then becomes water vapor in the atmosphere in the form of clouds (Yin process). When the water in the atmosphere cools, it undergoes a process called condensation (even more of a Yin

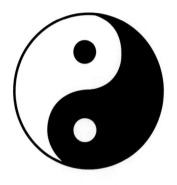

FIGURE 2-1 ■ Yin and Yang symbol.

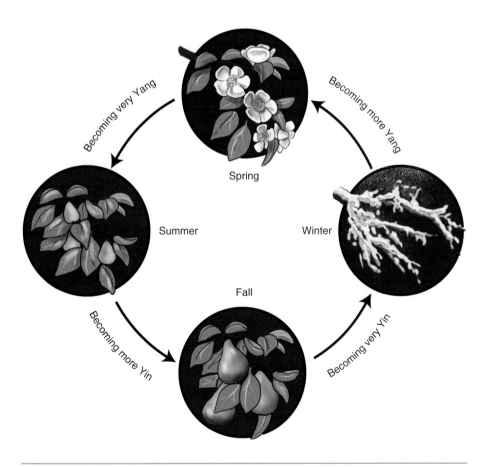

FIGURE 2-2 ■ Yin and Yang in the continuum of the seasons.

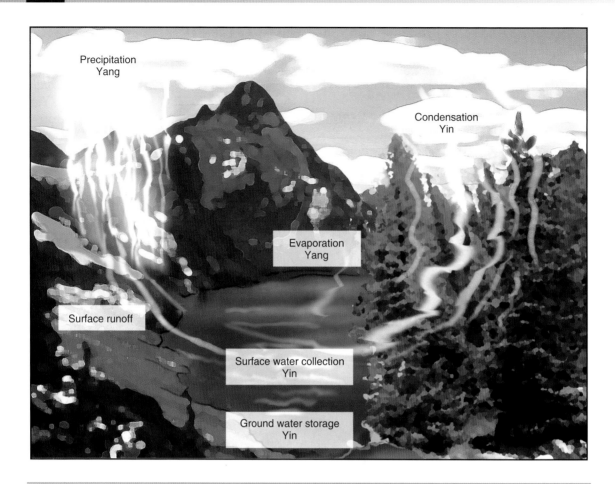

FIGURE 2-3 ■ Yin and Yang in the water cycle.

process) and becomes liquid, or rain. If the air is cold enough, the water will freeze into snowflakes or hailstones (a very Yin process). When raindrops, snowflakes, or hailstones become large enough and heavy enough, they fall from the clouds in the form of precipitation (a Yang process). Precipitation replenishes the Earth's water (Fig. 2-3).

The relationship between Yin and Yang can be used to realize the relationship among any structures, functions, and processes. The Yin characteristics of any of these are structure and substance; the Yang characteristics are activity and energy. For example, living creatures have form and mass, their Yin aspects. The ability to move, grow, and respond to changes in their environment is their Yang aspect (Table 2-1).

TABLE 2-1	Examples of Yin and Yang Phenomena
Yin Phenomena	**Yang Phenomena**
Cold	Heat
Rest	Movement
Passivity	Activity
Darkness	Light
Interior	Exterior
Contraction	Expansion
Decrease	Increase
Tranquil	Noisy
Static	Dynamic
Autumn and winter	Spring and summer
Night	Day
Female	Male

All the elements in Table 2-1 are opposite and complement of each other, yet they describe different aspects of the same phenomena. Again, remember that Yin and Yang can be considered in gradations of each other. The end of winter is more Yang than the dead of winter. The interior that is far from the surface is more Yin than the interior that is closer to the surface. The cool-down period of physical exercise is more Yin than the height of the physical exercise. Female is considered Yin, yet women have male hormones (called androgens that are responsible for, among other things, maintaining muscle and bone) that can be considered Yang. Males are considered Yang, yet they have an X chromosome, which can be considered Yin.

YIN AND YANG IN THE HUMAN BODY

The human body also has Yin and Yang aspects. In fact, all the metabolic processes that occur within the body can easily be seen as interplay between Yin and Yang. When blood sugar levels increase (a Yang activity), the pancreas secretes insulin to decrease the levels (a Yin activity). Digestion occurs in the gastrointestinal tract (interior, therefore a Yin aspect of the body), but digestive enzymes actively break down food, a Yang process. Hair and nails are solid structural parts of the body (Yin), but their growth involves dynamic cell division (Yang) (Table 2-2).

Again, remember that Yin and Yang are on a continuum. Even though metabolism is Yang, because it is active it can be further subdivided into Yin and Yang aspects according to traditional Chinese medicine, as shown in Table 2-3.

QI

The interplay and interaction of Yin and Yang create Qi. According to traditional Chinese medicine, all matter in the universe is formed from Qi. What differentiates one thing from another is the nature or state of its Qi. In its purest form, it is wholly energy, or completely Yang. When Qi becomes more concentrated or slows down, it forms matter, or enters a Yin state. This concept is easier to grasp if Qi is thought of in terms of the transformative states of Yin and Yang.

Going back to the example of the Earth's water cycle, when water is in a liquid state, it is

TABLE 2-2	Yin and Yang Aspects of Body Structure
Yin aspects	**Yang aspects**
Feet	Head
Lower body	Upper body
Anterior surface of the trunk	Posterior surface of the trunk
Medial surfaces of the extremities	Lateral surfaces of the extremities
Bones	Skin
Internal organs	Muscles
Body fluids (e.g., blood, lymph, mucus, cerebrospinal fluid, saliva)	Energy (e.g., Qi, metabolism [formation of ATP, digestion, etc.], nerve impulses, the flow of blood, lymph)

ATP, Adenosine triphosphate.

TABLE 2-3	Yin and Yang Relations of Bodily and Metabolic Functions
Yin	**Yang**
Cooling	Warming
Relaxing	Activating
Contracting	Expanding
Anchoring	Transporting
Nourishing	Consuming
Moistening	Drying
Storing	Protecting

Reprinted from Beresford-Cooke C: *Shiatsu theory and practice: a comprehensive text for the student and professional,* ed 2, Edinburgh, 2003, Churchill Livingstone.

more Yin. The heat from the sun is powerfully Yang (an active process); it heats the Earth and water from the oceans, lakes, rivers, and streams and converts the water into an increased Yang form through evaporation. The water absorbs energy from the sun and changes from a liquid to a gas. Because of the coldness of the atmosphere, or Yin, the water vapor forms clouds through condensation (even more of a Yin process) and becomes liquid, or rain. The water releases energy and changes from a gas to a liquid. If the air is cold enough, snowflakes or hailstones form; the most Yin form of water is ice. The water has released even more energy and changed from a liquid to a solid. Yin Qi of the water is converted into Yang Qi of water vapor and then is converted back into Yin Qi of water. Energy is absorbed and released as water changes states. Qi can be thought of as energy. Qi, then, is the force behind water changing states.

In the body, Qi is both the source behind the formation of substances and structures and is the energy and movement of substances and structures. Qi is the source of blood (Yin) and force behind the circulation of blood (Yang). Qi is the source of muscle (Yin) and energy required to make the muscle contract (Yang). Qi is the source of the nerves of the body (Yin) and the power driving nerve impulses (Yang). Substance structure, energy, and movement support each other; one cannot occur without the other.

QI, ORGANS, AND CHANNELS

Long before Western science had an understanding of the structure and function of the human body, the ancient Chinese had developed insight into the interrelations of Qi and the **organs**. Through thousands of years of experience, using both hands-on techniques and intuition, they came to a comprehension of the flow of Qi in the body as a system of channels (also called meridians). Qi in the channels is connected to organs of the body and is the living force that causes the organs to function. The organs have specific physiologic functions that are remarkably similar to the functions of organs in Western science, as well as emotional and spiritual correlations.

The organs in traditional Chinese medicine are Lung, Large Intestine, Stomach, Spleen, Heart, Small Intestine, Kidneys, Urinary Bladder, Liver, Gallbladder, Triple Heater (also called Triple Warmer or Triple Burner), and Heart Protector (also called Heart Constrictor or Pericardium). The channels connected to the organs have the same names: Lung Channel, Large Intestine Channel, and so forth.

All the organs are divided into Yin and Yang pairs (Table 2-4). Each pair belongs to one of the Five Elements (discussed in detail in Chapter 3).

In a perfect world, all living beings would have Yin and Yang in balance and smooth flow of

TABLE 2-4	Element Organ Pairs	
Yin organ	**Yang organ**	**Element**
Lung	Large Intestine	Metal
Kidney	Urinary Bladder	Water
Spleen	Stomach	Earth
Liver	Gallbladder	Wood
Heart	Small Intestine	Fire
Heart Protector	Triple Heater	Assisted Fire

Qi. Most human beings are born with a full and an equal amount of both. Various experiences in life such as emotional upset, physical trauma, illness, childbearing, and stress, to name a few, can cause blockages in the even flow of Qi. Asian bodywork therapies are designed to balance the flow of Qi. Specifically, shiatsu works by balancing the flow of Qi in the organ channels. Later chapters explain the techniques shiatsu practitioners use.

"All of life is a constant education."
~Eleanor Roosevelt

VITAL SUBSTANCES

Traditional Chinese medicine views the human body as more than just the sum of its parts. The study contains a definite understanding of the physiologic function of substances, tissues, and organs in the body as well as an awareness of metabolism. In addition, an appreciation of the emotional, spiritual, and metaphysical aspects of living beings is also a component. This appreciation is formulated from the ancient Chinese understanding of cycles of life and connection to the forces of the universe.

The physiologic and metabolic aspects of the body are considered as relationships and interactions among Vital Substances. The **Vital Substances** are Qi, **Blood**, **Essence** (**Jing**), and **Body Fluids**. Homeostasis depends on the amount and quality of these substances. They need to interact smoothly, and they need to support each other, or else the body will not function properly. Some of these are physical substances, such as **Blood**, Body Fluids, and Essence. They serve to nourish,

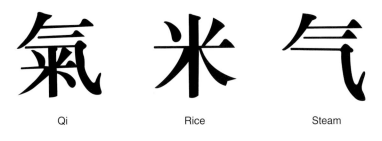

Qi   Rice   Steam

FIGURE 2-4 ■ Kanji characters for Qi.

moisten, and sustain the body, which are Yin activities. Another concept, **Shen**, refers to the mind or spirit. Shen and Qi bring the body to life and maintain vitality, which are Yang activities. All the other Vital Substances are simply manifestations of Qi.

QI

As previously mentioned, Qi is multidimensional. It is the energy behind the formation of the material and is energetic. For example, it is the force behind the formation of the wiring electricity travels along, as well as the flow of electricity itself. Even though "energy" is the most common translation of Qi, Qi has physicality as well. It can be sensed and palpated, and its flow can be changed through human-to-human connection. The Chinese character for Qi has two components: one for "rice" and one for "steam." In its metaphysical form, Qi dances and flows like the steam. When Qi slows and condenses, it brings forth the material, like rice (Fig. 2-4).

Qi has many roles in the body. It is the force behind movement, is the source of warmth, protects human beings from factors in the external environment, and governs metabolism. It also is the basis for the emotional, psychologic, and spiritual aspects of being human. Qi is the driving force behind the transformations that occur, such as moving from one emotional state to another, or absorption of nutrients from inside the digestive tract into the blood.

Source Qi is the basic form of Qi in the body, which is composed of a combination of three other forms: the Essential Qi of the Kidney; Qi of food, derived through the transformative function of the Spleen; and air (Great Qi) drawn in through the Lungs. Source Qi serves to energize all the organs, including the organs that helped create it, and it is the basis of all physical activity. All forms of Qi in the body are derivatives of Source Qi. It reaches the entire body through the pathways of San Jiao (Triple Heater Channel; see Chapter 3). The Triple Heater Channel is the "messenger of Source Qi" because all the other channels connect to it and receive their stock of Qi from it by a source point.

The Triple Heater Channel (San Jiao) is also known as the Triple Burner Channel or the Triple Warmer Channel. It is named for the three "heaters" (burners or warmers) of the body. The Upper Heater includes the functions of the Lungs and Heart. It receives air (Great Qi), which combines with the Qi of food; Source Qi acts as a catalyst for this process. The Middle Heater is where food is processed into food Qi by the functions of the Spleen and Stomach. Source Qi acts as a catalyst for this. The Middle Heater is sometimes referred to as a "bubbling cauldron." The Lower Heater includes the functions of the Large Intestine, Small Intestine, Urinary Bladder, and Kidneys. Its purpose is to separate the pure from the impure and eliminate waste; it acts like a drainage ditch. Source Qi also helps with this process.

Defensive Qi is a highly active Qi that protects the body from external pathogens and other harmful influences from the external environment. Defensive Qi (**Wei Qi**) is sent out by the Lungs and flows more toward the surface of the body (between muscles and the skin).

BLOOD

In traditional Chinese medicine Blood is more than the actual physical substance. It is a liquid form of Yin. Blood flow follows Qi flow; Qi flow follows Blood flow. "Qi is the leader of Blood; Blood is the mother of Qi" (from *The Yellow Emperor's Classic of Internal Medicine*). The purpose of Qi is expansive (Yang); it warms the body and causes movement of the entire body, a body part, or metabolism. Blood, on the other hand, nourishes body tissues and organs and is cooling, soothing and hydrating, all Yin properties. Blood is formed in the Heart, with the support of the Qi of food sent upward by the Spleen. The Liver stores the blood during times of relaxation and dispatches it to where it is needed during increased levels of activity.

Blood also has emotional and spiritual meanings. The Shen is the mind and/or spirit. It is the responsibility of Blood to soothe, calm, and provide respite for the Shen. If this does not occur, a restless mind that can lead to worry and insomnia may occur. Because the Liver is a storage depot and distribution center for Blood, a healthy Liver is related to healthy emotional and spiritual states.

ESSENCE (JING)

Source Qi is the Yang expression of Qi; it is the energy of movement and transformation. Yin Qi expression is Jing, which is usually translated as Essence. It is the foundation of the body's physicality. There are three types of Jing: Prenatal Essence, Postnatal Essence, and **Kidney Essence**.

Prenatal, or **Congenital**, **Essence** is responsible for the genetic physical **constitution** of the body. This is why children have body shapes and facial features similar to their ancestors. Prenatal Essence is present from conception and is stored between the Kidneys. One way to think of it is that each person is born with a certain amount of Prenatal Essence, which is the supply for life. It gradually decreases over time and cannot be re-created. Because its purpose is to provide the physical bodies of the next generation, both sexual activity and childbearing draw from Prenatal Essence.

Postnatal, or **Acquired**, **Essence** is produced from food by the Spleen and Stomach. Postnatal Essence travels to all other parts of the body to support them and to the Kidneys, where it is stored. A healthy diet and fitness level (to both strengthen the body and provide good breathing) can contribute to the formation of Postnatal Essence, and a temperate lifestyle can preserve it.

Both Prenatal and Postnatal Essence is part of Kidney Essence, which supports the Yin of the entire being. Kidney Essence circulates all over the body.

BODY FLUIDS

The most Yin of all body substances are the Body Fluids, which are supported by Kidney Yin. The Body Fluids include cerebrospinal fluid, synovial fluid, serous fluid, mucus, urine, tears, sweat, lymph, and blood. Blood, however, is so important that it is considered in its own domain. The clear and more dilute fluids are thought to travel in the exterior of the body, feeding the muscles and skin. The more viscous fluids circulate deeper and nourish the joints, central nervous system, eyes, nose, ears, and mouth.

Body Fluids are obtained from food and drink taken in by the body. In a complex operation, they are processed by the Spleen (using Source Qi from the Kidneys), the Kidneys, the Small Intestine, the Large Intestine, and the Urinary Bladder. The processing results in "pure" fluids that are sent to the Lungs to hydrate them and the muscles, skin, joints, central nervous system, and sense organs to moisturize and nourish them. The "impure" fluids leave the body in the urine and feces. The Triple Burners (or Heaters) are essential to the conversion and delivery of the Body Fluids.

SHEN

As previously stated, the Shen is most closely translated as the mind and/or spirit. It is the most metaphysical (or rarefied) and quintessential of the Vital Substances. It is intangibility itself. Because the body cannot live without the mind or the spirit, though, it is inextricably linked to the corporeal being and therefore linked to Qi and Essence. Shen gives the person his or her sense of self, also known as consciousness. The ability to form thought, have emotions, connect to others and surroundings, appreciate beauty, form a code of ethics, choose how to live, create new works, and have ideas that have never been thought of before are all aspects of Shen.

Although Shen is an abstract concept, it nonetheless has real manifestations. It can be reflected in the eyes, heard in the speech, and noticed in how a person carries himself or herself. The spirit of a person is infused in every fiber of his or her being. The Shen is said to reside in the Heart. Shiatsu, and all bodywork, has at its core the Shen.

CAUSES OF DISEASE

As previously stated, traditional Chinese medicine views the human body as an integral part of its surroundings and the universe. Human beings have a connection to nature and its cycles, ebbs, and flows. Those same cycles are within the body as well. The Yang of day warms and moves Qi. The Yin of night encourages Blood to cool, moisten, and nourish the tissues. This is also how traditional Chinese medicine views health—as flowing along a continuum. Thus, when the body is not in good health, disharmony is present in Qi flow. The shiatsu practitioner, using his or her own Qi, supports the client and helps restore the smooth flow of Qi. This can help the client's healing process and facilitate health maintenance.

The disruptions in Qi flow can be caused by many factors. These factors are grouped under three categories: Internal Causes (emotions), **External Causes** (weather), and other causes.

Internal Causes of Disease

There are six **Internal Causes of disease**; all are mental and/or emotional issues. These causes are joy, worry, sadness (and grief), anger, fear, and severe fright (shock). Joy, sadness, anger, and fear are associated with specific organs and the Qi of that organ. The corresponding organs or channels of each of the mental and emotional factors are outlined in Chapter 3.

Although all these are normal, natural states, they can lead to Qi imbalances. If the emotion was experienced suddenly and excessively, or if the emotion is experienced long term and never adequately expressed, it can cause disease. Chinese medicine recognizes that emotion is a part of human life and only causes disharmony if it is consistently repressed or experienced in the extreme. The Qi in the associated organ or channel is then affected in particular ways (Table 2-5).

Joy is centered in the Heart and serves to soothe the mind and Qi. Heart Protector does

| TABLE 2-5 | Effect of Emotions on Organs and Channels |

Emotion/mental state	Effect	Primary organs/channels affected
Joy	Slows Qi down	Heart
Panic	Scatters Qi	Heart
Worry	Knots Qi	Spleen and Lungs
Sadness (and grief)	Dissolves Qi	Lungs
Anger	Makes Qi rise	Liver
Fear	Descends Qi	Kidney
Severe fright (shock)	Scatters Qi	Kidney and Heart

just that—protects the Heart. It helps maintain emotional stability by being the "minister of the Heart" and the protector of Shen. Too much excitement and passion can disturb the mind and Shen. Therefore excessive excitement can injure the Heart by slowing down Qi relating to it. Excess joy in the form of mania often scatters the Qi.

Worry is associated with the Spleen, which is related to thinking, learning, and nourishment. Worry is basically the mind churning; it will not release an issue or calm down for much-needed rest. Worry can also knot the Qi of the Lungs and can be seen physically as the chest muscles constrict and breathing is hampered.

Sadness (and grief) particularly affects the Lungs, by way of the Heart, thereby serving to "dissolve" Qi. Sadness primarily affects the Heart, and the Lungs suffer in consequence because the Heart and Lungs are in the Upper Burner of the Triple Heater Channel. Sadness and grief can have a profound effect on the body, causing it to draw inward. The chest area can feel heavy and breathing can become difficult because these emotions deplete Qi in the Lungs.

Anger is under the Liver's purview. One of the Liver's purposes is to distribute emotional and physical Qi for evenness of energy and emotions. Anger causes a rise in Liver Yang; this is also known as "blazing of Liver Fire." If anger is not expressed and is instead turned inward, over time it can cause depression, and the Qi can then become stagnant.

Fear is related to the Kidneys and can cause Kidney Yin deficiency, or a deficiency of Essence.

One of the functions of the Kidneys is to give a person the ability to summon up energy when needed. Fear, though, descends the Qi, which can result in the paralysis that fear sometimes generates. Severe fright (shock) is the deeper form of fear that goes along with emotional trauma and physical injury. Qi is scattered. The Kidneys can easily become drained, and the Heart is disturbed because the mind needs to deal with the shattering experience.

External Causes of Disease or Pernicious Influences

Disharmonies within the body are likened to climatologic changes. The body is constantly being challenged by outside influences, such as pathogens, toxins, and mechanical injury. If the internal environment is out of equilibrium or the Defensive Qi is fragile, a person is at risk for the invasion of **Wind**, **Cold**, **Heat**, **Summer Heat**, **Damp**, and **Dryness**. These are also known as the Six Excesses. Each of these external conditions can then cause similar conditions internally.

The internal expressions of climate can also arise if the Qi of certain organs is inadequate. This makes it easier for external climates to invade. If an internal climate is already brewing, the external climate exacerbates the condition by ensconcing itself in the body and disrupting the associated organ's functioning. Onset is typically slow, and the conditions become chronic.

Wind. A saying in traditional Chinese medicine states, "A thousand evils ride on the wind." Wind is the predominant Qi of spring. The Wind can be from the atmosphere, or from artificial wind pathogens such as fans, air conditioning, open windows, and so forth. Wind creates movement in the body where there should be stillness; even the symptoms of Wind can move around within the body. Wind is the forerunner of other **pernicious influences**, and it usually teams up with the others to create **Wind-Cold**, **Wind-Heat**, or **Wind-Damp**. The main organs and channels affected by wind are the Liver and Gallbladder.

Wind-Cold has a sudden onset and is usually a common cold or flu. Early symptoms include fatigue and headache. They can develop into a mild fever, stuffy nose that has a runny, clear discharge, body aches, and cough. Chills are also present. Sometimes Wind-Cold transforms into Wind-Heat.

Wind-Heat also has a sudden onset, but with a fever rather than chills. The affected person has a stuffy nose with a yellow, sticky discharge, some body aches, a sore throat, cough, headache, and fatigue. These are all classic signs of the flu.

Wind-Damp is similar to Wind-Heat in that it manifests as a stomach flu or nausea. However, it can penetrate the joints and develop into arthritis. It can also cause muscle aches and soreness that travel around the body.

Internal Wind starts with a Liver issue and can gradually develop into tremors, seizures, a stroke, or Alzheimer's disease.

Cold. Cold is a contracting and freezing force. It is the predominant Qi of winter. Qi will slow and possibly stop moving, which causes pain. The body's metabolism slows, and the body becomes underactive. The person will crave warmth and have chills and shivering. Examples of Cold invasion are cold hands and feet, abdominal pain, pain and contraction of tendons, and aversion to cold. The person has a desire for warmth and warm drinks and foods. Examples of extreme Cold invasion are hypothermia and frostbite. Wind-Cold, as previously described, is the sudden onset of a common cold. The main organs and channels affected by cold are the Urinary Bladder and Kidneys.

Internal Cold is caused by a Yang deficiency. It can also be caused by overeating iced foods and drinks.

Heat. With Heat the body feels hot, and a fever can be present. It often occurs in summer but can occur in other seasons as well. The fluids concentrate and become yellow, and sweating occurs. Heat creates more thirst and sweat. Movement of Qi is sped up, but it is restless movement. Localized heat can be caused by localized infections characterized by redness, pain, heat, and swelling. The main organs and channels affected by heat are Heart, Heart Protector, Small Intestine, and Triple Heater.

Internal Heat can result from any issue involving Qi stagnation. As the Qi stagnates, it creates Heat. Heat also occurs from living in hot climates and overeating hot foods.

Summer Heat. Summer Heat only occurs in summer. The main clinical symptoms are headache, aversion to heat, sweating, thirst, and dark, scanty urine. Summer heat may also cause hyperthermia such as heat cramps, heat stroke, and heat exhaustion. The same organs and channels affected by Heat are affected by Summer Heat.

Damp. Damp is wet, heavy, slow, and turbid. It is the predominant Qi of late summer. Dampness can be caused by external factors such as a damp house or damp weather, or it can be caused by internal factors such as Qi stagnation due to lack of exercise. The main characteristics of dampness in the body are heaviness in the head and body, stickiness, conditions that are difficult to get rid of, and repeated attacks of symptoms. It lingers and descends in the body, causing joint problems, swelling, fullness in the chest and abdomen, diarrhea, and fatigue. The organs and channels affected by damp are the Stomach and Spleen.

When Exterior-Damp, caused by external factors, invades the body, it invades the legs first and then gradually moves upward through the leg channels and may settle in the pelvis. If this happens, it may endanger the reproductive organs.

Wind-Damp has as its main symptoms itchy skin, urticaria, sweating, body aches, feeling of heaviness, and swollen joints. **Damp-Heat** can appear as a vaginal infection or prostate inflammation, which is accompanied by fever. It is most frequent in summer and late summer. **Damp-Cold** can obstruct the Lungs, as in bronchitis. Internal Dampness is generated by a weak Spleen and sometimes Kidneys. **Internal Dampness** differs from External Dampness in that the clinical manifestations develop gradually rather than suddenly. Lack of exercise can be a cause because it slows down the Qi. Exercise moves the Qi and rids the body of stagnation. Diet plays a significant role in Dampness. Old, cold food (such as leftovers), canned food, foods high in fat, dairy products, excessive meat intake, and fried foods all create Dampness. Fresh food is much better for the body.

Dryness. Dryness is caused by a dry environment, dry wind, or dry indoor heating. It is the predominant Qi of autumn. It is a Yang pathogenic factor that tends to injure Yin or Blood. It dries the mucous membranes and causes thirst and constipation. The main organs and channels affected by dryness are the Lungs and Large Intestine.

Internal Dryness comes from Yin deficiency of the Stomach and/or Kidney. Because the Stomach is the origin of fluids, eating late at night, following an irregular diet, or becoming active right after eating can deplete stomach fluids and increase Dryness in the body.

Other Causes of Disease

Several other causes of disease were identified by the ancient Chinese. They include **weak constitution**, **overexertion**, **underexertion**, **excess sexual activity**, **bad diet**, **trauma** (injury), **parasites** and **poison**, and **incorrect treatment**. Although many advancements in both Eastern and Western medicine have occurred, these causes of disease are still prevalent today. Perhaps the context in which these factors occurred has changed, but their effects have not.

Weak Constitution. A person's constitution, or physical makeup, is determined by genetic factors, prenatal care and nutrition, and events surrounding birth. Traumatic illnesses and injuries can diminish the body physically and deplete Source Qi. Unhealthy habits also deplete the body and cause harm to it. If a person has a weak constitution, he or she is more susceptible to pernicious influences and illnesses.

Overexertion. Activity consumes Qi; rest restores Qi. Activity, whether mental or physical or both, depletes Spleen Qi and Kidney Qi. If recovery time is not long enough, these two organs are not able to replenish their Qi and a systemic illness may occur. If just one part of the body is excessively used (e.g., the elbow of a carpenter who swings a hammer with the same hand all day), Qi can become stuck in that area.

Underexertion. Lack of physical activity and mental activity causes a decrease in the circulation of Qi. This will weaken the function of the Spleen and Stomach and decrease the body's resistance to disease.

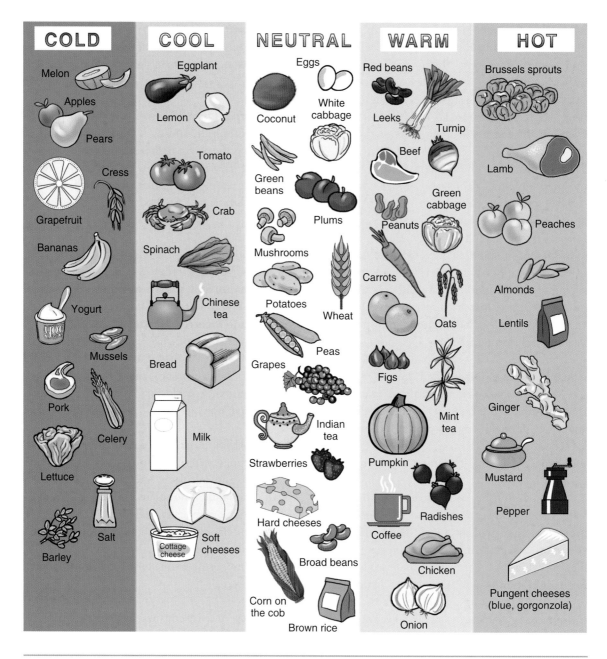

FIGURE 2-5 ■ Energetic properties of foods. (Adapted from Beresford-Cooke: *Shiatsu: theory and practice*, ed 2, Edinburgh, 2003, Churchill Livingstone.)

Excess Sexual Activity. What is considered excess sexual activity is different for each person. It depends on age, constitution, and amount of sexual activity. For men, ejaculation is a loss of Essence. Women tend not to lose as much Essence during sex. However, both men and women can deplete their Kidneys through too many orgasms. If recovery time is not adequate, Essence and Kidney Qi will not be rejuvenated.

Bad Diet. Eating foods that are processed, overeating one particular type of food, eating under stress or because of stress, and eating too quickly can all contribute to illness in the body. In particular, overeating foods that are cold, raw, sweet, and high in fat can injure the Spleen and Stomach. Eating fresh foods and a balance of different types of food is best (Fig. 2-5).

Trauma. Physical, mental, and emotional trauma cause stagnation of Qi and Blood. The stagnation can show up in different organs and tissues, such as chronic headaches, tight muscles, and digestive disorders and, in some cases, is quite painful. Even though traumas can heal, many years later the person can still be vulnerable to other pernicious influences.

Parasites and Poisons. Quite a variety of parasites can infect human beings: athlete's foot, malaria, hookworm, and so forth. Parasites drain the body's resources. Poisons come from a variety of sources—ingested chemicals, pollutants, and radiation. All of these can still weaken a person's constitution and make him or her vulnerable to illness.

Incorrect Treatment. Incorrect treatment is what it sounds like—the wrong treatment for a particular condition. This can happen in any type of treatment, Eastern or Western. For example, the wrong herbs can be prescribed for a particular condition, or the wrong medication given. In shiatsu it could mean incorrect application of techniques and resulting in harm to the client. Whether it be traditional Chinese medicine or modern Western medicine, if a person's condition is incorrectly treated, the original problem is not only not solved, it may perhaps lead to worse ones.

1. Draw a picture that represents the interrelationship of Yin and Yang.

2. Give five examples of Yin in the world and five examples of Yang in the world. Use examples other than the ones listed in the chapter.

Yin	Yang
_____	_____
_____	_____
_____	_____
_____	_____
_____	_____

3. List the Vital Substances and their functions in the human body.

4. Explain what Shen is.

_____

_____

_____

_____

5. For each of the following emotions, list its effect on Qi and what organs or channels are affected.

Emotion/Mental State	Effect	Primary Organs or Channels Affected
Joy	_____	_____
	_____	_____
Panic	_____	_____
	_____	_____
Worry	_____	_____
	_____	_____
Sadness (and grief)	_____	_____
	_____	_____
Anger	_____	_____
	_____	_____
Fear	_____	_____
	_____	_____
Severe fright (shock)	_____	_____
	_____	_____

6. For each of the following external causes of disease, list how they would present in the body. Also list recommendations that could be useful to someone who has this condition.

	Presentation in the Body	Recommendations
Wind-Cold	_____	_____
	_____	_____
	_____	_____

Wind-Heat _____ _____

_____ _____

_____ _____

Wind-Damp _____ _____

_____ _____

_____ _____

Internal Wind _____ _____

_____ _____

_____ _____

Cold _____ _____

_____ _____

_____ _____

Heat _____ _____

_____ _____

_____ _____

Summer Heat _____ _____

_____ _____

_____ _____

Damp _____ _____

_____ _____

_____ _____

Damp-Heat _____ _____

_____ _____

_____ _____

Damp-Cold _____ _____

_____ _____

_____ _____

Dryness _____ _____

_____ _____

_____ _____

7. Choose one of the other causes of disease. Write a paragraph on what causes it, how it presents in the body, and what recommendations could be given to someone who has it.

8. Think of an illness you have had and describe it in terms of traditional Chinese medicine.

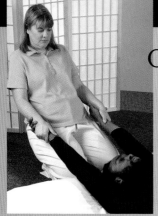

CHAPTER

3

FIVE ELEMENT THEORY

OBJECTIVES

Upon completion of this chapter, the reader will have the information necessary to do the following:

1. Describe the origin of the Five Elements.
2. List the correspondences for each of the Five Elements.
3. List the components of the Creation Cycle and explain how the Creation Cycle works.
4. Explain how the Control Cycle works.
5. Determine which of the Five Elements is personally predominant and explain why.
6. For each of the organ channels, list its functions, what it is related to in the body, what it symbolizes, its purposes according to traditional Chinese medicine, and whether it is Yin or Yang.
7. Describe the location of each organ channel on the body.
8. Palpate the location of each organ channel on the body.
9. List and explain the functions of key classic tsubo for each organ channel.
10. List the tsubo that are contraindicated in a pregnant client.

A s the ancient Chinese developed their philosophies and view of themselves in the larger scheme, they began to perceive their environment and the universe in ways other than just in terms of Yin and Yang. The manifestations of Qi revealed themselves to be ordered in five different manners, which have been translated as **Elements**, **Phases**, or **Transformations**. Phase and Transformation are terms that are closer to the literal translation of the concept from Chinese. Phase and Transformation are words that have change inherent in their meaning, which is part of what defines Qi. Qi is also defined by its different characteristics as it changes states in each of the Five Phases or Transformations. The word *Element* does not, perhaps, best represent this insight. However, Element is the more commonly used term and the one this text uses.

Assisted Fire (Lesser Fire, Supplemental Fire)
Control Cycle
Creation Cycle
Earth
Fire
Five Elements (Phases or Transformations)
Gallbladder
Heart
Heart Protector (Pericardium, Heart Constrictor)
Key Classic Tsubo
Ki
Kidney
Large Intestine
Liver
Lung
Metal
Small Intestine
Spleen
Stomach
Triple Heater (Triple Warmer, Triple Burner, San Jiao)
Urinary Bladder
Water
Wood

Ki is the Japanese word for Qi. Qi has been used in this text up to this point because the material covered has been related to traditional Chinese medicine. From this point on, however, more connections will be made between Chinese theory and shiatsu, which has Japanese origins. Therefore Ki will be used instead of Qi. Remember, though, that Qi and Ki mean the same thing.

Five Element Theory provides a useful foundation for beginning shiatsu practitioners. Ki is relatively easy to see in natural cycles reflected in the practitioner's own Ki and the Ki of his or her clients. Because shiatsu practitioners contact and work with a client's Ki, Five Element Theory provides a framework for understanding Ki, and differentiating its many qualities.

FIVE ELEMENT CYCLES

In traditional Chinese medicine, natural phenomena were systemized into Five Elements: **Metal**, **Water**, **Earth**, **Wood**, and **Fire**. Seasons, foods, flavors, colors, and sounds were categorized into each of the Elements. These became so ingrained in their way of life that through times of cultural upheaval in China, as people sought ways to find meaning and organization in their world, they used the Five Element Theory as a point of coordination. Soon just categorization of events and objects was not enough for Chinese people to understand their world. A deeper comprehension of the evolution, interaction, and metamorphosis of events and objects developed.

The interaction and relations among features of the universe, the environment, and the people became more important than mere classifications. The Five Elements were seen as a part of a cycle. The cause and progression of illnesses and disorders were perceived to be based on patterns of transformation within the cycle. Lack of health was seen to be caused by a lack of harmony among certain Elements. Ancient medicine expanded Five Element Theory to include aspects of the body: organs, sense organs, tissues, emotions, and behavioral attributes. Everything categorized under the Five Elements is referred to as correspondences; these correspondences were used as a reference for traditional Chinese medicine physicians in their practice of diagnosis and treatment (Fig. 3-1).

CREATION CYCLE

The **Creation Cycle**, also known as the Generation Cycle, Promoting Cycle, or Nurturing Cycle, is shown in Figure 3-2. This cycle is called the Creation, Generation, Promoting, or Nurturing Cycle because each Element supports, develops, and nourishes the Element that follows it (indicated by arrows), much as a mother nourishes a child. Earth supports Metal; metals form within the earth. Metal supports Water; metals are minerals and as such, they leach into springs, creating mineralized water. Water supports Wood; trees need water to grow. Wood supports Fire; wood is fuel for fire. Fire supports Earth; the ashes from fire fortify the soil, and earth is made from cooled magma.

The Five Elements continually generate and control each other, helping keep balance in the cycle. As an Element is being generated by its "mother," it is drawing and mixing with its Ki.

	Metal	Water	Earth	Wood	Fire
Season	Autumn	Winter	Late Summer	Spring	Summer
Direction	West	North	Center	East	South
Color	White	Black, Blue	Yellow, Brown	Green	Red
Taste	Pungent	Salty	Sweet	Sour	Bitter
Odor	Rotten	Putrid	Fragrant	Rancid	Burnt
Climate	Dryness	Cold	Dampness	Wind	Heat
Development Stage	Harvest	Storage	Transformation	Birth	Growth
State	Quieting	Slumber	Transition	Awakening	Wakefulness
Spiritual Quality	Po (Corporeal Soul; Body; Material)	Zhu (Ambition; Will)	Thought and Ideas	Hun (Ethereal soul; immaterial)	Shen (Spirit; awareness)
Yin Organ/Time of Day	Lungs 3 - 5 am	Kidneys 5 - 7 pm	Spleen 9 - 11 am	Liver 1 - 3 am	Heart 11 am - 1 pm
Yang Organ/Time of Day	Large Intestine 5 - 7 am	Urinary Bladder 3 - 5 pm	Stomach 7 - 9 am	Gallbladder 11pm - 1 am	Small Intestine 1 - 3 pm
Sense Organ	Nose	Ears	Mouth	Eyes	Tongue
Tissue	Skin and Body Hair	Bones	Muscles	Sinews	Vessels
Emotion	Sadness; Grief	Fear	Pensiveness	Anger	Joy
Sound	Crying	Groaning	Singing	Shouting	Laughing

FIGURE 3-1 ■ Five Element Correspondences.

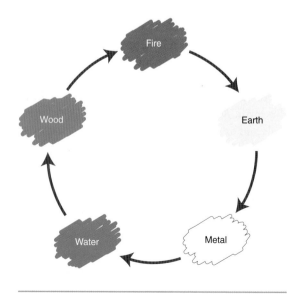

FIGURE 3-2 ■ Creation (Generation) Cycle.

This keeps an Element from expanding out of control and keeps its mother in balance. Along with this concept, if an Element has a particular imbalance, the imbalance is passed on to the next one. For example, if Wood does not nourish Fire, then Fire can become deficient. Both Wood and Fire would need to be addressed and rebalanced.

CONTROL CYCLE

A **Control Cycle** is also built into the Five Elements (Fig. 3-3). Along with the inherent control in the Creation Cycle (just described), each Element actively controls another. This compensatory mechanism exists to restrain imbalances in the Creation Cycle. Earth controls Water by absorbing water, and earthen dams keep water in check. Metal controls Wood; metal can cut

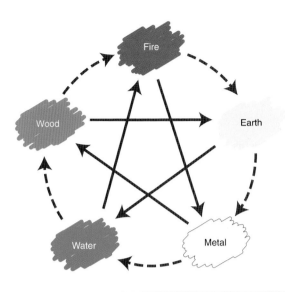

FIGURE 3-3 ■ Controlling Cycle.

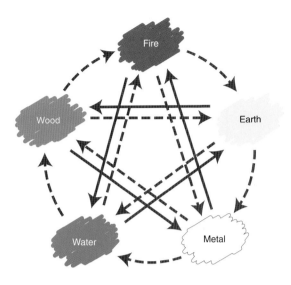

FIGURE 3-4 ■ Insulting Cycle.

through wood. Water controls Fire; water puts fire out. Wood controls Earth; trees are planted to prevent soil erosion, and plant roots can break through earth and rock. Fire controls Metal; fire heats metal so it can be shaped.

If an Element becomes deficient, or imbalanced, it is not able to manage the Element it is responsible for controlling. That Element then becomes disproportionately strong. It may, in fact, becomes so strong that it turns around and "insults" its controlling Element. The cycle then becomes severely out of balance, and multiple Elements would need to be addressed to restore equilibrium (Fig. 3-4).

FIVE ELEMENT "TEST"

All persons have aspects of all the Five Elements within them. To have a better understanding of the Five Elements and how they relate to "real life," a "test" can be taken to see which is predominant. Even though someone may be mainly one Element, other Elements may be prevalent in different aspects of his or her life. For example, someone may be mainly Wood in his or her professional life but keeps his or her home the way an Earth does. This test is meant as a tool for insight, not necessarily as a guide for how to live life (Fig. 3-5).

ORGAN CHANNELS

A complete understanding of the channels that belong to each Element is essential to the practice of shiatsu. Tables 3-1 to 3-5 provide descriptions of each of the Elements, their correspondences, their functions, their symbolic representations, and their functions according to traditional Chinese medicine. Also included are descriptions and diagrams of the channel locations on the human body and key classic points (tsubo). Key classic points are fixed tsubo that the shiatsu practitioner may find helpful to address for particular client issues. Listed with the points are the English meanings of the point in quotes followed by the Chinese name of the point.

PREGNANCY

Working tsubo on pregnant clients involves special considerations. During pregnancy, the fetus uses quite a bit of the mother's Ki and Blood while it is growing. Before delivery, the mother's Ki and Blood should be supported and the mother's Ki "lifted." Working certain tsubo is contraindicated in pregnant women because these tsubo have a strong "down bearing" effect on Ki. These are **Large Intestine** (LI) 4, **Spleen** (SP) 6, **Stomach** (ST) 36, and **Gallbladder** (GB) 21.

If a pregnant woman is past her due date, then working these points may be useful in stimulating the downward flow of Ki and possibly starting labor and delivery.

Check all that seem to describe you. Be honest! At the end of each section, total the number you have checked under each lettered section. The letter code for the Five Elements is at the end of the "test." The section you have the most checks in is the element you have the most of.

A

_____ Cautious and sensible

_____ Keep my feelings, thoughts and opinions to myself; careful what I reveal to others

_____ Like privacy over intimacy, solitude over socializing

_____ Like intellectual pursuits

_____ Like to figure things out for myself

_____ Am objective and unemotional

_____ Feel self-sufficient in or out of a relationship

_____ Am skeptical, even cynical

_____ It's easy for me to adapt to new situations

_____ Am patient and will persevere, even against the odds

_____ Strongly prefer or dislike salty foods

_____ Strongly prefer or dislike the colors blue or black

_____ Strongly prefer or dislike winter

_____ Often dream of lakes, rivers, oceans or dark, mysterious places

_____ Am prone to ear problems – loss of hearing, ringing in the ears, ear aches, ear infections

_____ Often feel excessively thirsty

_____ Am prone to urinary problems

_____ Hair falls out easily, or have thinning hair or baldness

_____ Extremely high energy or total depletion between 3 p.m. and 7 p.m.

_____ **TOTAL for A**

FIGURE 3-5 ■ Five Element test.

B

_____ Am confident and assertive about my abilities

_____ Bullheaded and stubborn

_____ Tend to be competitive and a workaholic

_____ Comfortable leading or directing others

_____ Have creative solutions to difficult problems

_____ Am direct and straightforward, sometimes to the point of being insensitive

_____ Sometimes I have trouble controlling my anger

_____ Fear losing control and being helpless

_____ Trust my own instinct about what is right and wrong

_____ Like to be recognized for my talents and achievements

_____ Strongly prefer or dislike sour foods

_____ Strongly prefer or dislike the color green

_____ Strongly prefer or dislike windy conditions

_____ Often dream of forests, growing plants, trying to reach a goal

_____ Have dry, red, itchy or teary eyes, or blurred vision

_____ Fingernails and toenails split, peel and crack easily

_____ Have chronic headaches or migraines

_____ Have chronic tension in my neck and/or shoulders

_____ Restlessness or difficulty sleeping between 11 p.m. and 3 a.m.

_____ **TOTAL for B**

FIGURE 3-5, cont'd ■ Five Element test.   _Continued_

C

_____ Intuitively know what others are thinking and feeling

_____ Sometimes laugh too loud, too much or inappropriately

_____ Like laughter and joy in my life

_____ Tend to wear my emotions on my sleeve

_____ Either flourish or crumble in stimulating environments, like a big city or noisy office

_____ Am animated, enthusiastic and full of life

_____ Scatterbrained and absent-minded

_____ Am vulnerable, especially in relationships

_____ Other people seem to be drawn to me

_____ Love sensual pleasures

_____ Need a lot of support and praise

_____ Strongly prefer or dislike bitter foods

_____ Strongly prefer or dislike the color red

_____ Strongly prefer or dislike very hot climates

_____ Often dream of romantic relationships or sexual encounters

_____ Have spontaneous sweating, hot flashes or a tendency to overheat

_____ Prone to varicose veins, hemorrhoids or problems involving blood vessels

_____ Have heart palpitations, especially when excited or stressed

_____ Extremely high energy or totally depletion between 11 a.m. and 3 p.m.

_____ **TOTAL for C**

FIGURE 3-5, cont'd ▦ Five Element test.

D

_____ Like tranquil settings and natural beauty

_____ Conflict upsets me easily

_____ Am nurturing and like to take care of others

_____ Tend to put others' needs before mine

_____ Tend to eat when I'm lonely or uncomfortable

_____ Difficult for me to ask for what I need

_____ Like feeling full – with food, friends, social engagements, but sometimes feel weighed down or overstuffed

_____ Like being the center of my social network

_____ Set unrealistic expectations and sometimes am disappointed in how things turn out

_____ Tend to worry, be obsessive or compulsive

_____ Strong preference or dislike for sweet foods

_____ Strong preference or dislike for the color yellow

_____ Strong preference or dislike for damp climates

_____ Often dream of houses, backyards and grassy fields

_____ Gain weight easily and find it difficult to lose weight

_____ Have frontal headaches, usually due to worrying

_____ Prone to indigestion, abdominal pain or excess stomach acid

_____ Prone to blood sugar issues – diabetes or hypoglycemia

_____ Extremely high energy or totally depletion between 7 a.m. and 11 a.m.

_____ **TOTAL for D**

FIGURE 3-5, cont'd ▪ Five Element test.

Continued

E

_____ Like doing puzzles, solving riddles and reading mysteries

_____ Like to make lists to create order in my life

_____ Tend to be neat and orderly in my personal appearance

_____ Tend to be stiff and formal in social situations

_____ Able to resist temptation

_____ Don't like to get caught up in others' dramas

_____ Strongly committed to certain moral principles and standards of conduct

_____ Enjoy using logic and analytical approaches to solve problems

_____ Dislike crowds, waiting in lines, traffic lights, etc.

_____ Like organization in myself and others

_____ Don't express my feelings; sometimes I'm called unemotional or unfeeling

_____ Strong preference or dislike for pungent and spicy foods

_____ Strong preference or dislike for the color white

_____ Strong preference or dislike for very dry climates

_____ Often dream about mountain peaks, snow or the interiors of boats, cars or trains

_____ Prone to hay fever or other nasal allergies

_____ Chronic sinus problems

_____ Problems with the bowels – diarrhea, constipation, or alternating between the two

_____ Restlessness, agitation or high energy between 3 a.m. and 7 a.m.

_____ **TOTAL for E**

A – Water
B – Wood
C – Fire
D – Earth
E – Metal

FIGURE 3-5, cont'd ▪ Five Element test.

TABLE 3-1	Metal

Season:	Autumn
Direction:	West
Color:	White
Taste:	Pungent
Odor:	Rotten
Climate:	Dryness
Development stage:	Harvest
State:	Quieting
Spiritual quality:	Po (corporeal soul; body; material)
Yin organ/time of day:	Lungs/3-5 AM
Yang organ/time of day:	Large Intestine/5-7 AM
Sense organ:	Nose
Tissue:	Skin
Emotion:	Sadness, grief
Sound:	Crying

Lung Channel (LU; Fig. 3-6)
Yin Organ

Function:	Intake of Ki
Related to:	Nose, sinuses, throat, bronchii, lungs, skin, breathing
Symbolically represents:	Structure and vitality
	Boundaries
Traditional Chinese medicine:	Governs Ki and respiration
	Disperses fluids (mist fluids) and Wei Qi
	Descends Ki (prevents scattering and exhaustion of Ki)
	Regulates water passages
	Houses corporeal soul
Trunk/arm/hand:	Lung Channel begins at LU-1, which is approximately 1 inch inferior to the hollow under the lateral end of the clavicle. From there it travels through the most anterior portion of deltoid, biceps brachii, and over brachioradialis. It then runs down the lateral aspect of the anterior (Yin) arm, where the skin is fairer and thinner. It proceeds along the inside of the tendon of brachioradialis, over the wrist onto the pad of muscle on the thumb side of the palm (Big Fish) to finish at LU-11, on the tip of the radial side of the edge of the thumbnail.

Key Classic Tsubo

LU-1	"Central treasury," *Zhongfu*
	Located approximately 1 inch inferior to the hollow under the lateral end of the clavicle. This point clears fullness, phlegm, and fluids from the chest. It can also relieve pain in the upper chest and back and stop coughing.
LU-5	"Cubit marsh," *Chize*
	Located in the most lateral depression of the elbow crease, on the Yin side of the arm. It clears phlegm, Heat, and Cold from the Lungs and helps the Lungs descend Ki and fluids.
LU-7	"Broken sequence," *Lieque*
	Located in a depression approximately 1 inch from the end of the wrist crease, on the lateral edge of the radius, proximal to the styloid process. This point releases grief and tension and is excellent for stimulating the body's defense (Wei Qi) because it causes sweating.
LU-9	"Great abyss," *Taiyuan*
	Located at the lateral end of the wrist crease in the depression lateral to the radial artery. It tonifies the Lung Ki in the chest and influences circulation. It is useful for weakness and chronic lung troubles.

Continued

TABLE 3-1	Metal—cont'd
LU-10	"Fish border," *Yuji*
	Located halfway along the radial edge of metacarpal I. This point relieves a painful sore throat.
LU-11	"Lesser metal," *Shaoshang*
	Located on the tip of the radial side of the edge of the thumbnail. It stimulates the diffusion and descent of Lung Ki, benefits the throat, promotes breathing, and expels exterior Wind.
Large Intestine Channel (LI; Fig. 3-7)	
Yang Organ	
Function:	Elimination
Related to:	Large intestine, mouth, throat, nose, mucous secretions, bowel movements, secretions
Symbolically represents:	Ability to release
Traditional Chinese medicine:	Descends its Ki
	Allows passage of waste
Hand/arm:	LI starts at LI-1, located on the radial side of the nail of the index finger. It travels on the posterior (Yang) arm along extensor digitorum and extensor carpi radialis, then along the anterior edge of brachioradialis. It runs up between the two heads of biceps brachii, through anterior deltoid to LI-15 on the acromioclavicular joint.
Shoulder/neck:	From the acromioclavicular joint LI travels over the top of the shoulder, then diagonally along the anterior neck, through the center of sternocleidomastoid. It approaches the face at the jaw, just anterior to the ramus of the mandible.
Face:	LI follows the "smile line" to the lateral border, ending at LI-27, outside the nostril on either side of the nose.
Key Classic Tsubo	
LI-1	"Metal Yang," *Shangyang*
	Located on the thumb side of the index finger's nail. This point clears Heat, brightens the eyes, helps the ears and throat, expels Wind and scatters Cold, and removes blockages in the channel.
LI-4	"Union valley," *Hegu*
	Located on the highest point of the web of flesh between the thumb and metacarpal II, when the thumb is adducted. ⚠ **This point is not to be used on a pregnant client.**
	This is the main point for the face, especially for frontal headaches, toothaches, and sinusitis. It is often effective at stopping pain.
LI-10	"Arm three li," *Shousanli*
	Located in the most lateral depression in the elbow crease on the Yang side of the arm. It clears phlegm, Heat, and Cold from the Lungs and helps the Lungs descend Ki and fluids. Removes obstructions from the channel. Major point for treating any muscular problems of the forearm and hands.
LI-11	"Pool at the bend," *Quchi*
	Located at the lateral end of the elbow crease, halfway between LU-5 and the lateral epicondyle of the humerus. This point is effective for Heat trapped in the upper body: sore throats, infections, itchy skin, breakouts and rashes, and so forth. It also tones the body, cools the Blood, and expels Exterior Wind.
LI-20	"Welcome fragrance," *Yingxiang*
	Located on the outside lateral part of the nostril in the nasolabial groove. This point treats disharmonies caused by Exterior Wind: facial paralysis, hay fever, the common cold, and so forth.

⚠ = Caution.

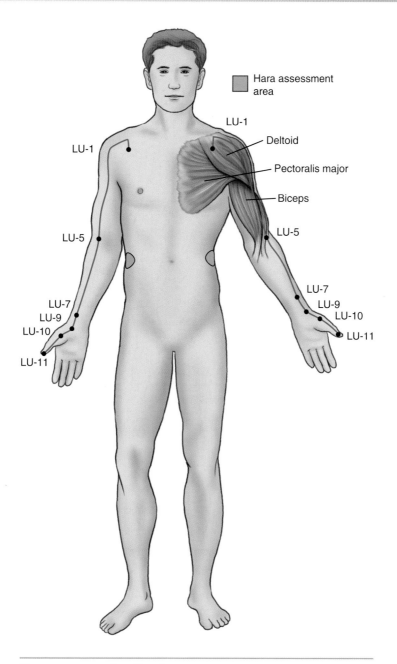

FIGURE 3-6 ■ Lung Channel.

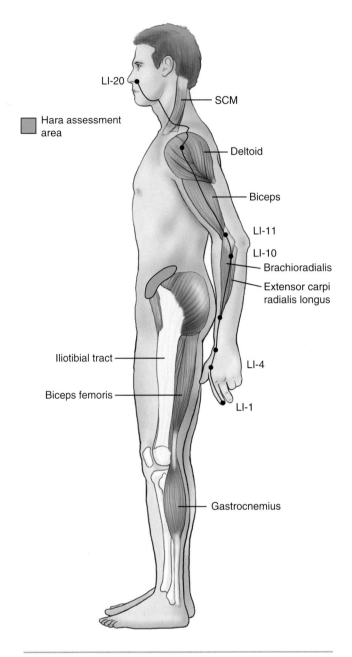

FIGURE 3-7 ■ Large Intestine Channel.

TABLE 3-2   Water

Season:	Winter
Direction:	North
Color:	Black (blue)
Taste:	Salty
Odor:	Putrid
Climate:	Cold
Development stage:	Storage
State:	Slumber
Spiritual quality:	Zhi (ambition, will)
Yin organ/time of day:	Kidneys/5-7 PM
Yang organ/time of day:	Urinary Bladder/3-5 PM
Sense organ:	Ears
Tissue:	Bones
Emotion:	Fear
Sound:	Groaning

Kidney Channel (KI, Fig. 3-8)
Yin Organ

Function:	Water metabolism, controls all fluid secretions, governs endocrine system, impetus.
Related to:	Kidneys, pituitary gland, adrenals, stress response, fear and phobias, sexual hormones, desire for reproduction, ears, bones and lower back.
Symbolically represents:	Impetus, flexibility, ability to respond to stimulus, ability to summon up energy when needed.
Traditional Chinese medicine:	Houses the essence.
	Stores fundamental Yin and Yang of the body.
	Governs water.
	Grasps or anchors Lung Ki.
	Produces marrow; brain and the central nervous system
	Houses willpower and ambition.
Foot/leg:	Kidney begins at KI-1 ("bubbling spring"). This is on the plantar surface of the foot, where the ball of the foot meets the instep, in the hollow between metatarsals I and II.
	KI then ascends along the medial side of the foot, angling posteriorly and proximally to KI-3 on the superior surface of the medial malleolus, just anterior to the Achilles tendon. KI circles posteriorly around the medial malleolus to KI-6 on the inferior surface of the medial malleolus. From there, KI ascends the lower leg by moving proximally up the medial head of gastrocnemius to the medial side of the popliteal fossa, where the tendons of semimembranosus and semitendinosus meet. KI continues along the medial surface of the upper leg, just posterior to the adductors, to where the inguinal region joins the perineum. At this point, KI travels internally.
Trunk:	KI emerges on the abdomen immediately superior to the pubic crest and approximately $\frac{1}{2}$ inch from the midline of the body. KI runs superiorly on the thorax, widening to follow the lateral edges of the sternum. It terminates at KI-27, in the hollow inferior to the medial end of the clavicle.

Continued

TABLE 3-2	Water—cont'd

Key Classic Tsubo

KI-1	"Bubbling spring," *Yongquan* Located on the plantar surface of the foot, where the ball of the foot meets the instep, in the hollow between metatarsals I and II. Relieves headaches and dizziness, tonifies Yin, clears Heat, calms Shen (spirit), restores consciousness.
KI-3	"Greater stream," *Taixi* Located in the depression between the tip of the medial malleolus and the Achilles tendon. Source point; directly benefits the kidney organ. Tonifies Yin and Yang of the entire body, regulates the uterus, tonifies the lower back and knees.
KI-6	"Shining sea," *Zhaohai* Located approximately ½ inch directly below the tip of the medial malleolus. Benefits Yin and fluids, clears Heat in the Blood, tonifies the uterus, relieves insomnia as it calms the Shen. Relieves throat problems.
KI-27	"Transporting point mansion," *Shufu* Located in the hollow inferior to the medial end of the clavicle. This point promotes the descent of Lung Ki, stops coughing, harmonizes the stomach, and stops vomiting.

Urinary Bladder Channel (UB, Fig. 3-9)
Yang Organ

Function:	Governs autonomic nervous system, energy supply of all organ functions, transformation of fluids, and purification of Ki.
Related to:	Will, determination, intensity, fatigue, fear, uterus, urinary bladder, spine, bones, fluid balance, reproduction.
Symbolically represents:	Impetus, ability to respond, purification, fluidity.
Traditional Chinese medicine:	Tonifies all the organ functions. Receives impure fluids from Kidneys and transforms them into urine. Stores and excretes urine. Influences uterine function. Influences posture by giving strength and support to the back.
Head/neck:	UB starts at UB-1 in the hollow superior to the inner canthus of the eye and, bilaterally, travels superiorly to the forehead. It widens slightly at the superior portion of the frontal bone then travels over the top of the head, then down the posterior of the head to the occipital ridge. It travels down the posterior cervical region approximately 1 inch lateral to the vertebral column.
Trunk:	UB continues from the neck down the back in two lines. One branch travels laterally and inferiorly along the medial border of the scapula and then approximately 2 inches lateral to the vertebral column to the level of the fourth sacral foramina. The other branch continues in a straight vertical line through the erector spinae muscles to the lowest sacral foramina. It then ascends to the top of the sacrum to descend again more medially and diagonally over the sacral foramina to the end of the coccyx.

TABLE 3-2	Water—cont'd

Hip/leg/foot:	The two branches of UB continue through the posterior leg and meet in the center of the popliteal fossa at UB-40. The medial branch travels laterally through the gluteals to the center of the transverse gluteal fold. It descends through the center of the posterior thigh. It veers laterally for the last third of the posterior thigh to the lateral side of the popliteal fossa, then goes to the center of the popliteal fossa to UB-40. The lateral back branch continues from the lowest sacral foramina along the lateral curve of the gluteal muscles. It angles slightly medially and crosses the other posterior thigh branch of UB about a hand's width superior to the popliteal fossa. It descends inferiorly to UB-40. UB then descends distally down the middle of gastrocnemius, and travels laterally to pass between the Achilles tendon and the lateral malleolus. It curves around the lateral malleolus then travels along the lateral edge of the foot to end at UB-67, on the lateral side of the little toe's toenail.
Key Classic Tsubo	
UB-2	"Bamboo gathering," *Zanzhu*
	Located inferior to the medial end of the eyebrow, in the supraorbital notch. Relieves headache, blurred vision; tearing from exposure to the wind, twitching of the eyelids, redness, swelling of the eyes. Stops pain, soothes the Liver, removes blockage from the channel.
UB-10	"Celestial pillar," *Tianzhu*
	Located within the posterior hairline, along the suboccipital groove, approximately $\frac{3}{4}$ inch lateral to the midline of the posterior neck. Dispels Wind; dissipates Cold; relieves headache, stiff neck, and lower back pain; clears the brain; brightens the eyes.
UB-40	"Bend middle," *Weizhong*
	Located in the center of the transverse crease of the popliteal fossa. Clears the Blood, discharges Heat, relieves Wind-Dampness, treats lumbar pain and restricted movement of the hip joint.
UB-57	"Mountain support," *Chengshan*
	Located in between the heads of gastrocnemius, just proximal to the Achilles tendon.
	Cools and moves the Blood, relieves cramps and pain in the legs and knees, treats hemorrhoids and constipation, clears Summer Heat.
UB-60	"Kun Lun mountain," *Kunlun*
	Located in the depression between the Achilles tendon and the tip of the lateral malleolus. Relieves headache; stiffness in the neck, shoulders and arms; and back pain. Expels Wind, clears Heat and invigorates the Blood.

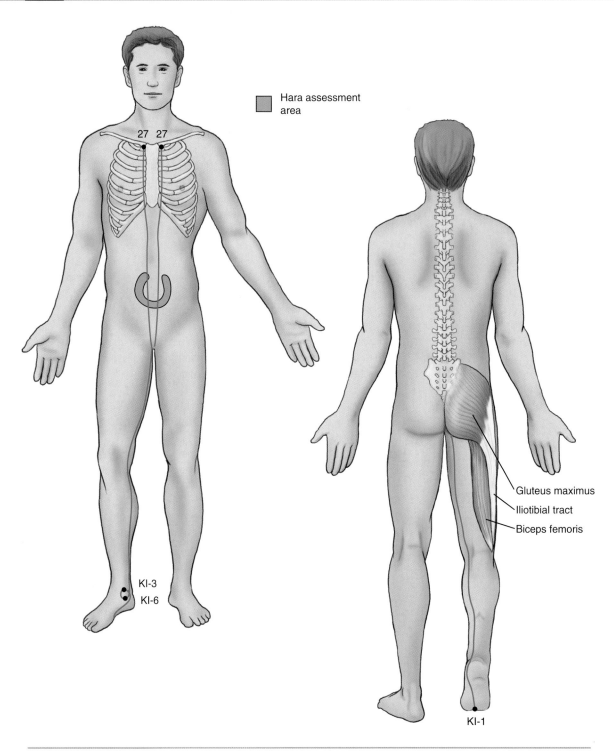

FIGURE 3-8 ■ Kidney Channel.

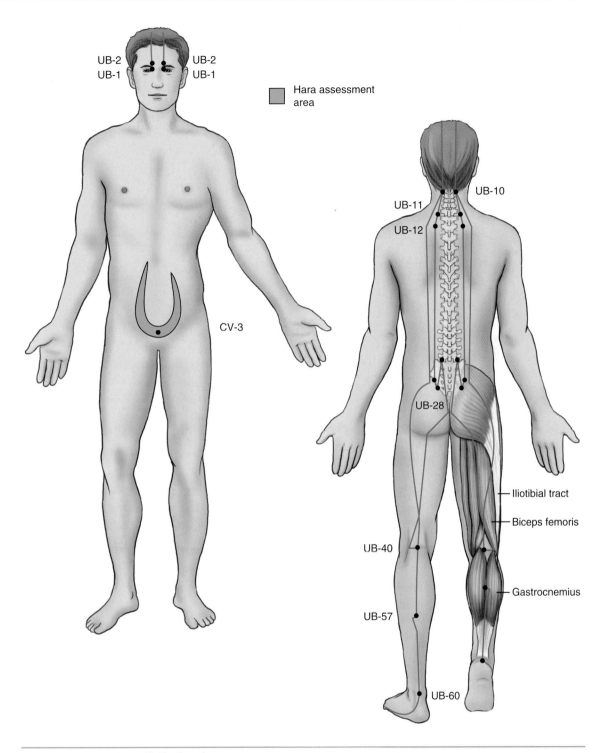

FIGURE 3-9 ■ Urinary Bladder Channel.

TABLE 3-3	Earth
Season:	Late summer
Direction:	Center
Color:	Yellow
Taste:	Sweet
Odor:	Fragrant
Climate:	Dampness
Development stage:	Transformation
State:	Transition
Spiritual quality:	Thought and ideas
Yin organ/time of day:	Spleen/9-11 AM
Yang organ/time of day:	Stomach/7-9 AM
Sense organ:	Mouth
Tissue:	Muscles
Emotion:	Pensiveness
Sound:	Singing

Spleen Channel (SP; Fig. 3-10)
Yin Organ

Function:	Digestive secretions, hormones.
Related to:	Thinking, pancreatic enzymes, saliva, stomach juices, insulin, glucagon, small intestine juices, bile.
Symbolically represents:	Nurturing, fertility, intellect, digestion of food and ideas, ability to think and learn, nourishment.
Traditional Chinese medicine:	Transforms and transports food and water (root of Postnatal Ki).
	Contains the Blood.
	Controls the muscles and the four limbs.
	Lifts or raises the Ki.
	Houses thought (thinking, studying, memorizing, analyzing).
Foot/leg/abdomen:	SP starts on SP-1 on the medial aspect of the big toe, approximately $1/16$ inch from the corner of the nail. It travels medially on the foot to SP-4 at the highest point of the longitudinal arch, then runs through the ankle, anterior to the medial malleolus. It travels proximally along the calf just anterior to gastrocnemius, past the medial border of the patella then through the conjunction of vastus medialis and rectus femoris into the inguinal region. SP then runs superiorly through the abdomen 1 inch lateral to the lateral border of rectus abdominis.
Trunk:	Just inferior to the rib cage, SP gently angles laterally to line up with the nipple, then travels superiorly through the nipple and pectoralis major to SP-20, which is approximately 1 inch inferior and slightly medial to LU-1. It then descends inferiorly and laterally to end at SP-21, which is located at the center of the axillary line and the level of the seventh rib space (approximately one hand width inferior to the axilla).

Key Classic Tsubo

SP-1	"Hidden white," *Yinbai*
	Located on the medial aspect of the big toe, approximately $1/16$ inch from the corner of the nail. Relieves Blood stagnation, helps contain the Blood, calms the Shen, and strengthens the Spleen.
SP-4	"Yellow emperor," *Gongsun*
	Located at the highest point on the longitudinal arch, in the depression distal to the base of metatarsal I. Supports the Spleen and the Stomach; relieves stomach and abdominal pain, vomiting and diarrhea; and stops bleeding.

TABLE 3-3	Earth—cont'd

SP-6	"Three Yin crossing (or intersection)," *Sanyinjiao*
	Located 2 inches directly proximal to the tip of the medial malleolus and $\frac{1}{2}$ inch posterior to the tibia. Circulates, cools, and nourishes the Blood; relieves Dampness; nourishes Yin; calms the Shen; promotes sleep; and assists the Spleen, Liver, and Kidney. It also assists in smoothing the flow of Liver Ki.
	⚠ **This point is not to be used on a pregnant client.**
SP-9	"Yin mound spring," *Yinlingquan*
	Located on the lower edge of the medial condyle of the tibia, in the space between the posterior border of the tibia and gastrocnemius. Relieves and removes Dampness, particularly of the lower heater.
SP-10	"Sea of blood," *Xuehai*
	Located 1.5 inches proximal to the medial and superior borders of the patella, on the bulge of vastus medialis. Removes blood stasis and cools and tonifies Blood.
SP-21	"Great embracement," *Dabao*
	Located at the center of the axillary line and the level of the seventh rib space (approximately one hand width inferior to the axilla).
	Regulates Ki and Blood; relieves pain in the chest, weak limbs, and asthma. Used to manage general pain from blood stasis.

Stomach Channel (ST; Fig. 3-11)
Yang Organ

Function:	Intake of food, transportation of nutrients, digestive tubes, governs overall appetites.
Related to:	Esophagus, stomach, duodenum, appetite mechanism, lactation, ovaries, uterus, menstrual cycle.
Symbolically represents:	Nurturing, fertility, groundedness (heartiness).
Traditional Chinese medicine:	Controls "rotting and ripening" of food ("bubbling caldron").
	Descends its Ki.
Face/throat:	ST begins under the center of the eye at ST-1 and travels down the cheek just past the corner of the mouth. It angles laterally to the jawline, then travels posteriorly along the mandible to ST-6 in the center of masseter. From there a branch ascends directly up to the superior edge of temporalis. ST continues inferiorly along either side of the esophagus to ST-9, then descends toward the head of the clavicle where it runs horizontally along the superior edge of the clavicle.
Trunk:	At the midpoint of the clavicle, ST descends to the nipple along the mammary line. At the level of the fifth rib, it angles gently toward the lateral edge of the rectus abdominis.
Abdomen/leg:	ST travels inferiorly along the rectus abdominis to just superior to the pubic bone, then angles diagonally across the inguinal line to the anterior, lateral edge of the rectus femoris, the lateral border of the patella, tibialis anterior.
Ankle/foot:	At the ankle, ST travels along the lateral edge of the tendon of the second toe and follows it distally to end at ST-45, on the lateral end of the toenail.

Key Classic Tsubo

ST-1	"Tear container," *Chengqi*
ST-2	"Four whites," *Sibai*
ST-3	"Great bone hole," *Juliao*
	Located in a vertical line down the cheek, centered under the pupil. ST-1 is at the midpoint of the infraorbital ridge; ST-2 is in the center of the infraorbital foramen; ST-3 is just under the maxilla. All brighten the eyes and face. ST-2 and ST-3 clear and disperse face swelling and pain, expel Wind, and reduce sinus problems.
ST-6	"Jaw vehicle," *Jiache*
	Located in the center of masseter, at the ramus of the mandible. It opens the jaw and relieves painful stiffness in the neck, expels Wind, and removes obstructions from the channel.

⚠ = Caution.

Continued

TABLE 3-3	Earth—cont'd
ST-9	"Man's prognosis," *Renying* Located at the anterior border of the sternocleidomastoid, level with the tip of the Adam's apple. This point relieves sore, and swollen throat, cough, and dizziness; and regulates Ki.
ST-21	"Beam gate," *Liangmen* Located approximately a hand's width above the navel, along the lateral edge of rectus abdominis. Regulates the Stomach, relieves belching (rebellious Ki), and stops pain.
ST-25	"Celestial pivot," *Tianshu* Located approximately 2 inches lateral to the center of the navel. Tonifies the intestines, clears Heat, and regulates Ki.
ST-30	"Surging Qi," *Qichong* Located on the upper border of the pubic bone along the edge of rectus abdominis. Removes stagnation of Ki and Blood in the lower heater, regulates Stomach Ki, promotes and nourishes essence, and stimulates digestive processes of the Stomach and Spleen.
ST-36	"Leg three mile," *Zusanli* Located approximately 2½ inches below the lower border of the patella, and ½ inch from the crest of the tibia. Tonifies Ki and Blood, expels Wind and Damp, increases Yang, and generally strengthens the lower body. It is a good point for any problems from the knee downward into the ankle and foot. It also increases the feeling of well-being. In fact, ST-36 is the most important of the more than 1000 points in the body and can be worked in any and all treatments. ⚠ **This point is not to be used on a pregnant client**.
ST-45	"Sick mouth," *Lidui* Located on the lateral end of the second toe's toenail. This point clears Heat in the Stomach, clears Heat from the channel, calms and opens the mind, and promotes breathing.

⚠ = Caution.

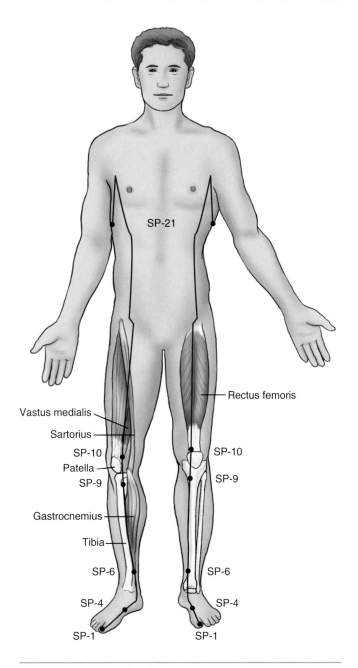

FIGURE 3-10 ■ Spleen Channel.

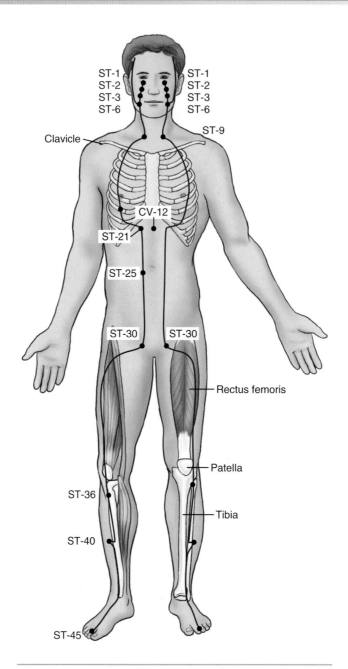

FIGURE 3-11 ■ Stomach Channel.

TABLE 3-4	Wood
Season:	Spring
Direction:	East
Color:	Green
Taste:	Sour
Odor:	Rancid
Climate:	Wind
Development stage:	Birth
State:	Awakening
Spiritual quality:	Hun (ethereal soul, immaterial)
Yin organ/time of day:	Liver/1-3 AM
Yang organ/time of day:	Gallbladder/11 PM-1 AM
Sense organ:	Eyes
Tissue:	Sinews
Emotion:	Anger
Sound:	Shouting

Liver Channel (LV; Fig. 3-12)
Yin Organ

Function:	Stores nutrients, controls the free flow of Ki throughout the body, governs detoxification and controls the blood.
Related to:	Ease of flow, control, detoxification, vision, eyes, tendons, nails, excessive behavior/overindulgence, energetic and emotional ups and downs, major decision making.
Symbolically represents:	Choice and execution of one's life plan, vision, planning, action.
Traditional Chinese medicine:	Gives capacity for being goal oriented, resolute, for having drive and energy.
	Hun rooted in the Liver.
	Ensures the smooth flow of Ki.
	Stores the Blood.
Foot/leg:	LV starts at LV-1, on the medial side of the big toe, $\frac{1}{16}$ inch from the corner of the toenail, and travels along the lateral aspect of the big toe's tendon to the anterior ankle. From there it runs along the medial edge of the tibia to approximately two thirds up the calf, then arcs gently up through the posterior-medial calf to approximately 1 inch inferior to the medial knee. LV then angles anteriorly for approximately 1 inch, then travels just under gracilis in the medial thigh to the pubis.
Abdomen/trunk:	From the pubis LV angles laterally and superiorly to LV-13, which is just inferior to the tip of the eleventh rib (floating rib). It continues to angle superiorly and medially to end on LV-14, which is on the mammary line between ribs 6 and 7.

Key Classic Tsubo

LV-1	"Big mound," *Dadun*
	Located on the medial side of the big toe, $\frac{1}{16}$ inch from the corner the toenail. This point helps regulate menstruation and promotes breathing.
LV-2	"Moving between," *Xingjian*
	Located at the base of the big toe just distal to the metacarpophalangeal joint.
	Aids in cooling the Blood, clearing Liver Fire, and calming Liver Yang. Useful for headaches, insomnia, painful eyes, and painful urination.

Continued

TABLE 3-4	Wood—cont'd

LV-3	"Supreme surge," *Taichong*
	Located on the dorsal surface of the foot, at the junction of metatarsals I and II. Source point of the Liver. Aids in the smooth flow of Liver Ki, roots Liver Yang. Relieves spasms, cramps, and headache. Calms the mind.
LV-8	"Spring at the bend," *Ququan*
	With the knee flexed, located at the medial end of the popliteal crease, just posterior to the medial condyle of the tibia, and the superior border of the tendons attaching to the medial aspect of the knee. It nourishes the Blood and clears Damp-Heat, especially from the lower burner. Locally, it is used to treat pain and swelling in the medial knee and upper leg.
LV-13	"Camphorwood gate," *Zhangmen*
	Located just inferior to the tip of the eleventh rib (floating rib).
	Relieves stagnation by promoting the smooth flow of Liver Ki. Harmonizes the Stomach and Spleen. Used to treat pain in the lower lumbar area and ribcage, spasms, abdominal distention, vomiting, diarrhea, hypertension, and excessive weight loss.
LV-14	"Cycle gate," *Qimen*
	Located on the mammary line between ribs 6 and 7.
	Cools the Blood, harmonizes the Stomach and promotes the smooth flow of Liver Ki. Useful for hiccups, vomiting, abdominal/thoracic tightness or distention, depression, mastitis, difficulty in giving birth, coughing, general body aches, and respiratory difficulty.
Gallbladder Channel (GB; Fig. 3-13)	
Yang Organ	
Function:	Controls digestive secretions, distributes emotional and physical Ki.
Related to:	Sides of the body, control of digestive secretions, eyes, tendons, flexibility, clarity in everyday decision making, discrimination and impartiality, ability to take risks versus timidity.
Symbolically represents:	Accomplishment, courage, spirit, gall.
Traditional Chinese medicine:	Stores and excretes bile.
	Controls judgment and decision making.
Head/neck:	From GB-1 at the lateral corner of the eye, GB descends posteriorly to the junction of the mandible and the earlobe. It then ascends anteriorly and superiorly to the middle of temporalis, descends straight down approximately 1 inch, then descends posteriorly to where the top of the ear attaches to the skull at Triple Heater (TH) 21. GB then ascends straight up approximately 1.5 inches, then descends the head, moving around the ear, and down to the mastoid process. GB then curves upward and anteriorly along the superior edge of temporalis to GB-14 in the forehead, which is approximately ½ inch above the eyebrow, in line with the pupil of the eye. GB then curves posteriorly back over the head approximately 1 inch more medial than where it curved up onto the head, then runs down to the occipital ridge, posterior to the mastoid process and attachment of upper trapezius. It descends the upper border of trapezius to the midpoint of the shoulder, where it goes internally.
Trunk:	GB reemerges below the axilla and angles inferiorly and medially to GB-24 on the eighth rib. It then travels almost straight posteriorly to GB-25 on the tip of the twelfth rib. From GB-25, GB again travels anteriorly along the anterior iliac crest to the anterior superior iliac spine.
Leg/foot:	From the anterior superior iliac spine, GB travels posteriorly to GB-30, located one third of the way between the greater trochanter and the sacrum. GB then angles anteriorly to descend the upper lateral leg along the iliotibial tract band, and the fibula in the lower lateral leg. Approximately one third of the way down the fibula, GB travels anteriorly in a straight line approximately 1 inch to GB-36, then angles inferiorly back to the fibula to catch the lateral tendon of the fourth toe. GB ends at GB-44, on the lateral side of the fourth toe, $\frac{1}{16}$ inch from the corner of the toenail.

TABLE 3-4	Wood—cont'd

Key Classic Tsubo

GB-1	"Pupil bone hole," *Tongziliao*
	Located in the indentation just lateral to the corner of the eye.
	This point relieves local eye pain, migraine headaches, and ankle pain along the channel at the lateral malleolus.
GB-14	"Yang white," *Yangbai*
	Located on the forehead approximately ½ inch above the eyebrow, in line with the pupil of the eye. It relieves exterior Wind, unilateral headaches, eye pain, vertigo, and various eye diseases.
GB-20	"Wind pond," *Fengchi*
	Located just under the occiput, in the hairline, between sternocleidomastoid and trapezius. Expels Exterior and Interior Wind, clears the mind, treats eye and ear pain and difficulties, and subdues Liver Yang.
GB-21	"Shoulder well," *Jianjing*
	Located on the mound of the shoulder, halfway between the neck and the acromion process. This point creates a strong downward movement and is helpful with relieving neck and shoulder stiffness and for treating many problems in child birthing. It brings the baby down in labor and delivery and promotes lactation in nursing mothers. ⚠ **This point is not to be used on a pregnant client.**
GB-25	"Capital gate," *Jingmen*
	Located on the posterior and lateral aspect of the torso, on the tip of the twelfth rib. It relieves pain in the hip joint, lower abdominal pain, abdominal urgency, asthma, dark urine, and diarrhea.
GB-30	"Jumping circle," *Huantiao*
	Located one third of the distance between the greater trochanter and the sacrum. It is the meeting point of UB and GB and helps decrease pain in the hip and pelvis. It also tonifies the Blood and Ki, relieves Damp-Heat in the groin and rectal area, treats influenza, and relieves sciatic pain.
GB-34	"Yang mound spring," *Yanglingquan*
	Located in the indentation that is anterior and inferior to the head of the fibula. It is useful in treating pain and swelling of the knee and relaxing the tendons. It also expels Wind from the knee and legs; clears Damp-Heat; treats constipation, lumbar pain, and numbness; and promotes the smooth flow of Liver Ki.
GB-40	"Hill ruins," *Qiuxu*
	Located in the indentation anterior and inferior to the lateral malleolus, lateral to the tendon of extensor digitorum longus. Source point for GB. Encourages smooth flow of Liver Ki. Useful for neck, axillary, and costal pain; pain and swelling of the lateral malleolus; abdominal pain; sighing; coughing; rapid breathing; and general body weakness. It strengthens Gallbladder's mental aspect, which enables the ability to make difficult decisions.
GB-44	"Yin orifice," *Zugiaoyin*
	Located on the lateral side of the fourth toe, $\frac{1}{16}$ inch from the corner of the toenail. This point subdues Liver Yang, clears Heat, brightens the eyes, and calms the mind.

⚠ = Caution.

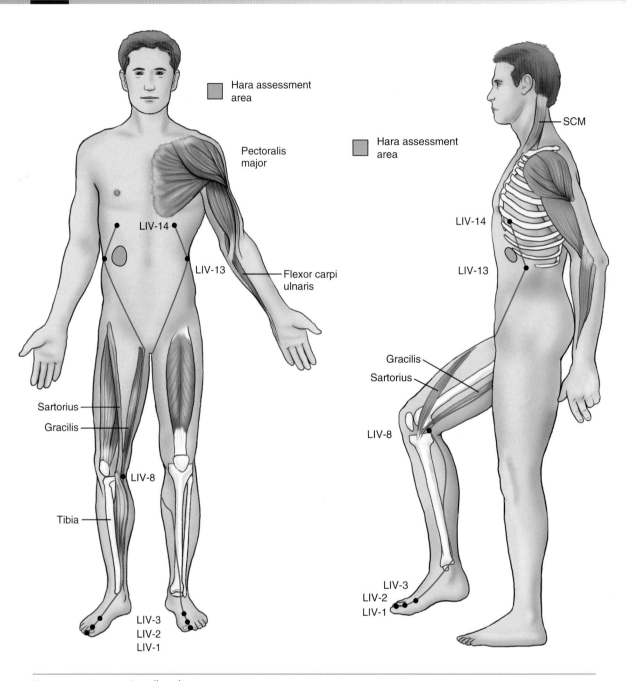

FIGURE 3-12 ■ Liver Channel.

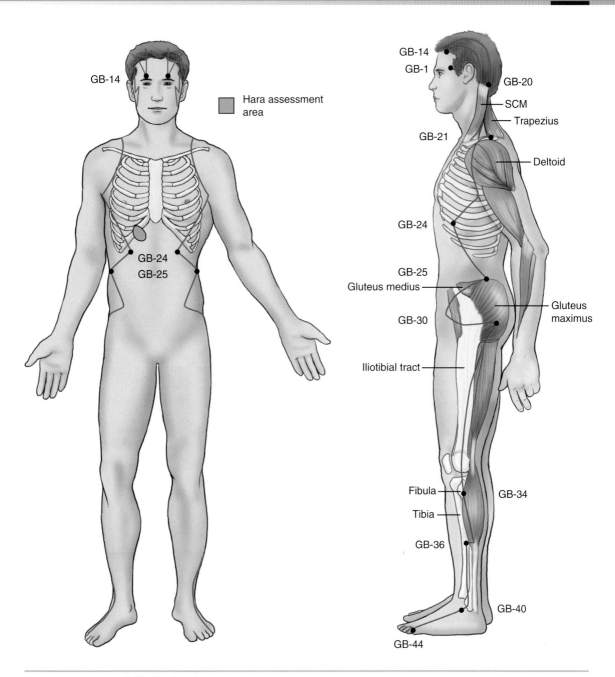

FIGURE 3-13 ■ Gallbladder Channel.

TABLE 3-5	Fire
Season:	Summer
Direction:	South
Color:	Red
Taste:	Bitter
Odor:	Burnt
Climate:	Heat
Development stage:	Growth
State:	Wakefulness
Spiritual quality:	Shen (spirit, awareness)
Yin organ/time of day:	Heart/11 AM-1 PM
Yang organ/time of day:	Small Intestine/1-3 PM
Sense organ:	Tongue
Tissue:	Vessels
Emotion:	Joy
Sound:	Laughing

Heart Channel (HT; Fig. 3-14)
Yin Organ

Function:	Adaptation, emotional Interpretation of experience.
Related to:	Heart, tongue, speech, sweat, complexion, central nervous system (brain), thymus.
Symbolically represents:	Emotional adaptation, emotional stability, spirit.
Traditional Chinese medicine:	Governs and propels the blood.
	Controls the blood vessels.
	Houses Shen.
	Controls sweat.
Arm/hand:	HT extends from HT-1, in the center of the axilla, out along the anterior (Yin) arm between biceps brachii and triceps brachii. It travels along the medial aspect of the ulna to end on HT-9, on the radial side of the little finger, $\frac{1}{16}$ from the corner of the nail.

Key Classic Tsubo

HT-1	"Utmost spring," *Jiquan*
	Located in the center of the axilla. It nourishes Heart Yin, opens the chest, stops pain in the chest and cold pain in the arm an elbow, and treats dryness of throat and nausea.
HT-3	"Lesser sea," *Shaohai*
	Located in the crease of the elbow in the depression anterior to the medial epicondyle of the humerus. Clears empty or full Heat from the Heart, calms the Shen, and removes obstructions from the channel, cardiac pain, depression, and dizziness.
HT-7	"Spirit's gate," *Shenmen*
	Located at the medial end of the wrist crease, in between the pisiform and hamate, on the radial side of the flexor carpi ulnaris. It tonifies the Heart and Blood, clears the mind, calms the Shen, and stops cardiac pain and hysteria.
HT-9	"Lesser Yin penetrating," *Shaochong*
	Located on the radial side of the little finger, $\frac{1}{16}$ inch from the corner of the nail. This point clears Heat, calms and opens the mind, extinguishes Wind, and promotes breathing.

Small Intestine Channel (SI; Fig. 3-15)
Yang Organ

Function:	Assimilation and absorption of food and experiences of all kinds.
Related to:	Small intestine, the spine, cerebrospinal fluid, shock mechanism.
Symbolically represents:	Assimilation (to convert another substance into ourselves), receiving, being filled, transforming.

TABLE 3-5	Fire — cont'd

Traditional Chinese medicine:	Separates the pure from the impure (digestive function).
Hand/arm/shoulder:	SI starts at SI-1, on the ulnar side of the little finger, $\frac{1}{16}$ inch from the corner of the nail. It travels through the medial wrist then along the posterior (Yang) side of the arm on the medial edge of the ulna ("on the border of the red and white skin"). It crosses through the elbow between the olecranon process and the medial epicondyle of the humerus. It travels up the arm through the center of triceps brachii and the axillary crease to SI-10 in an indentation just posterior to the acromion process.
Shoulder/back:	From SI-10, SI travels inferiorly and medially to SI-11 in the center of the scapula. It then ascends directly superior to SI-12 in the middle of supraspinatus. SI travels medially (and slightly inferiorly) to SI-13. From there it runs superiorly to C7.
Neck/head/face:	From C7, SI ascends diagonally across the neck and sternocleidomastoid to SI-17, just inferior to the earlobe. It then travels anteriorly and superiorly onto the jaw, just behind the ramus of the mandible, and up and under the cheek. It travels laterally and posteriorly back along the zygomatic arch to end at SI-19, in an indentation in front of the tragus of the ear.
Key Classic Tsubo	
SI-1	"Lesser marsh," *Shaoze*
	Located on the ulnar side of the little finger, $\frac{1}{16}$ inch from the corner of the nail. This point expels Wind-Heat, promotes breathing, removes blockages from the channel, clears Heat, and promotes lactation.
SI-3	"Back ravine," *Houxi*
	On a loose fist, this point is proximal to the head of the fifth metacarpal, on the medial side of the hand ("between the red and white skin"). SI-3 is the opening point for Governing Vessel (see Appendix), so it benefits the back and spine. It also eliminates Interior and Exterior Wind; promotes clarity of mind; and relieves headache, stiff neck and shoulder, and hypertonicity of the elbow, arm, and fingers.
SI-9	"Shoulder integrity," *Jianzhen*
	Located approximately 1 inch above the posterior axillary crease. It relieves pain in the shoulder blade, arm, and hand.
SI-10	"Scapula hollow," *Naoshu*
	Located in the depression just inferior and posterior to the acromion process of the scapula, directly above SI-9. It relieves pain and tonifies the shoulder and arm.
SI-11	"Celestial gathering," *Tianzong*
	Located in the center of the scapula. It is a key point to the back. It diffuses Ki stagnation in the chest and lateral ribcage.
SI-12	"Grasping the wind," *Bingfeng*
	Located in the suprascapular fossa directly above SI-11. It relieves pain and numbness in the shoulder, arm, and hand.
SI-19	"Palace of listening," *Tigong*
	Located between the temporomandibular joint and the tragus of the ear in the depression that occurs when the jaw is open. It relieves pain and boosts visual and hearing acuity.
Assisted Fire (Supplemental Fire, Lesser Fire)	
Yin organ/time of day:	Heart Protector (Heart Constrictor, Pericardium)/7-9 PM
Yang organ/time of day:	Triple Heater (Triple Burner, Triple Warmer)/9-11 PM

Continued

TABLE 3-5	Fire—cont'd

Heart Protector Channel (HP; Fig. 3-16)
Yin Organ

Function:	"Minister of the Heart," protects Shen, provides circulation for the inner core, governs the vascular system.
Related to:	Heart organ; deep/central circulation; function of the great blood vessels, veins, and arteries; blood pressure; vulnerability; inside/anterior surfaces.
Symbolically represents:	Emotional stability, messenger of the spirit/Shen by way of dreams, mother of Blood/ protector of Blood, defends the emotional core.
Traditional Chinese medicine:	Mediates with Source Ki on the level of consciousness by connection with the Heart and Shen. Energetic buffer zone around the Heart, protecting it from pernicious influences, shock, emotional trauma. Protects the Blood of the Heart, related to circulation of blood in the great vessels. Ensures stability of Shen, spreads influence of Shen throughout the body-mind. Works with Heart in ensuring a smooth flow of Ki and Blood in the chest and throughout the body.
Trunk:	HP starts at HP-1, which is found in the fourth intercostal space, just lateral and slightly superior to the nipple. It travels superiorly to the axilla.
Arm/hand:	Coming through the anterior axilla, HP travels along the anterior (Yin) arm between the heads of biceps brachii, then through the center of the elbow. From there it travels in between flexor carpi radialis and palmaris longus, and through the center of the palm to end at HP-9, on the radial side of the tip of the middle finger.

Key Classic Tsubo

HP-1	"Heavenly pond," *Tianchi* Located in the fourth intercostal space, just lateral and slightly superior to the nipple. This point relieves pain and swelling in the axillary region and pain in the stomach area.
HP-3	"Curved marsh," *Quze* Located inside the elbow crease, on the medial side of the tendon of the biceps brachii. It moves Blood stagnation, clears Heat in the Blood, relieves rebellious Stomach Ki, and is a revival/resuscitation point.
HP-6	"Inner border gate," *Neiguan* Located 1½ inch proximal to the transverse crease of the wrist, between the tendons of palmaris longus and flexor carpi radialis. This point connects with the Triple Heater (TH) Channel through TH-5, which is directly opposite HP-6 on the posterior arm. It opens the chest, relieving pain and stagnation; calms the Shen and relieves insomnia; releases the diaphragm and pacifies the stomach; and assists in treating hiatal hernia, nausea, and vomiting. It plays a key role in regulating Heart Ki and Blood.
HP-8	"Palace of labor," *Laogong* Located on the palm of the hand, between metacarpals II and III. It clears Fire in the Heart and eliminates Heat, relieving cardiac pain, mania, withdrawal, and epilepsy. It calms the Shen and treats and relieves vomiting, mouth sores, and bad breath.
HP-9	"Middle pouring," *Zhongchong* Located on the radial side of the tip of the middle finger. This point tonifies the channel and can relieve irritability, tinnitus, and vertigo.

TABLE 3-5   Fire—cont'd

Triple Heater Channel (TH; Fig. 3-17)
Yang Organ

Function:	Psychologic protection, peripheral circulation of blood and lymph, distributor of Source Ki and information between all organ systems, a warming force, feed system of Kidney Fire.
Related to:	Superficial and abdominal fascia/mesentery, blood circulation, lymphatic system, metabolism, immunity, infections, allergic reactions, thermoregulation, ears, deafness, swollen glands, tonsillitis, migraines, stiff neck and shoulders, skin, mucous membranes.
Symbolically represents:	Protection versus openness, emotional response to the process of creating physical and nonphysical boundaries, governs body surface, defends against pathogens or emotional insult.
Traditional Chinese medicine:	Facilitates free passage of or is an avenue for Source Ki.
	Three spaces in the body that need to be warm and allow for transformation:
	Upper burner: Lungs and Heart ("like a mist").
	Middle burner: Stomach, Spleen ("like a bubbling caldron").
	Lower burner: Kidney, Urinary Bladder, Small Intestine, Large Intestine ("like a drainage ditch"; involved in removing waste).
Hand/arm/shoulder:	TH starts at TH-1 on the tip of the ulnar side of the fourth finger, $\frac{1}{16}$ inch from the corner of the nail. It travels along the fourth finger's tendon and up the posterior forearm just to the medial side of the midline. TH then runs over the olecranon process, up through the center of the lateral head of triceps brachii, and through posterior deltoid to TH-14 at the acromion process. TH then travels medially along the supraspinatus.
Neck/head/face:	From TH-14, TH travels medially along the supraspinatus, then runs up the lateral border of trapezius to the occiput. From the most lateral edge of the occiput, TH branches anteriorly toward the face to under the earlobe. It circles laterally around the earlobe to where the earlobe attaches to the head, then rises superiorly to TH-22 on the most lateral aspect of the zygomatic arch. TH crosses in a straight line to end at TH-23 on the lateral end of the eyebrow.

Key Classic Tsubo

TH-1	"Gate/barrier rushing," *Guanchong*
	Located on the tip of the ulnar side of the fourth finger, $\frac{1}{16}$ inch from the corner of the nail. This point relieves headache, red eyes, sore throat, irritability, dry mouth, nausea and vomiting, arm pain, and pain in the fingers.
TH-4	"Yang pool," *Yangchi*
	Located in the wrist crease between the tendons of extensor digitorum and extensor digiti minimi. It is the source point for TH and thus tonifies the Source Ki of the entire body. It helps regulate menstruation, transforms fluids, and relieves Dampness from the lower burner. It also tonifies the stomach.
TH-5	"Outer gate," *Weiguan*
	Located $1\frac{1}{2}$ inch width proximal to the wrist crease in between the radius and the ulna. This point is directly opposite HP-6. It dissipates Wind; clears Heat and resolves toxins; benefits the ear; relieves Liver Yang aggravation, making it helpful for headaches, ear, and eye pain, and pain anywhere in the upper body.
TH-23	"Silk bamboo hollow," *Sizhukong*
	Located in the indentation at the lateral end of the eyebrow. This point dispels Wind and resolves Heat, clears and brightens the eyes, and relieves temporal headaches.

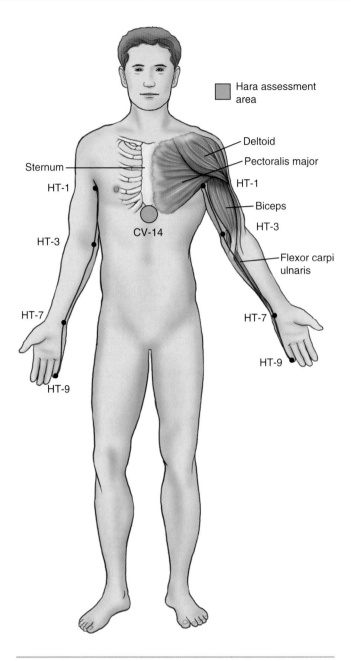

FIGURE 3-14 ■ Heart Channel.

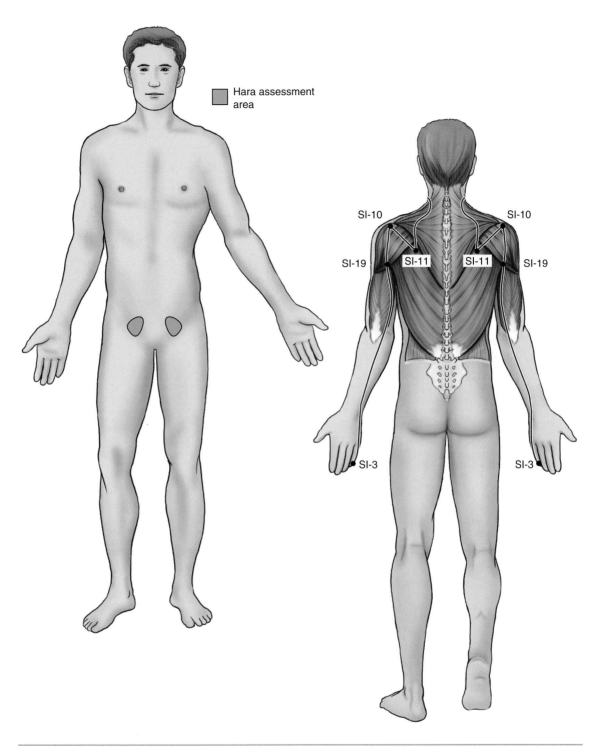

Hara assessment area

SI-10   SI-10

SI-19   SI-11   SI-11   SI-19

SI-3   SI-3

FIGURE 3-15 ■ Small Intestine Channel.

Continued

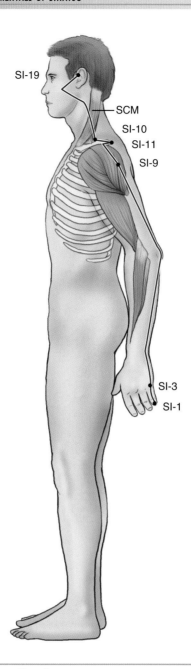

FIGURE 3-15, cont'd ▦ Small Intestine Channel.

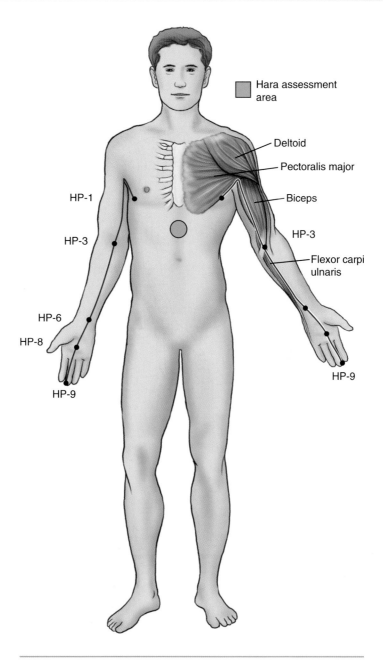

FIGURE 3-16 ■ Heart Protector Channel.

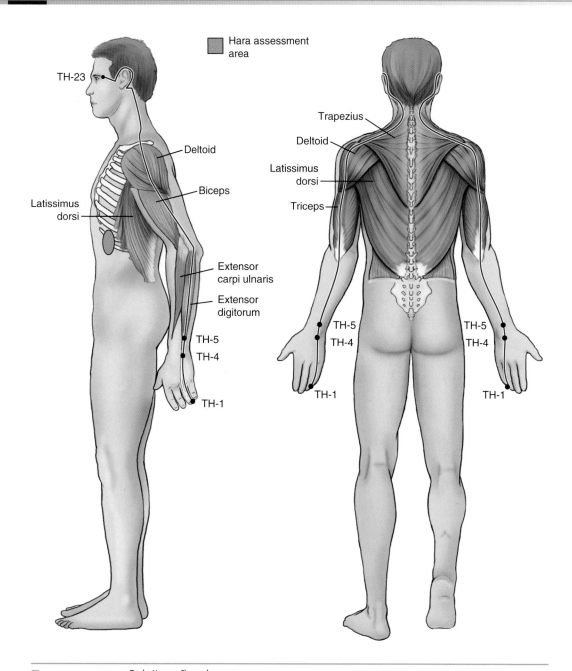

FIGURE 3-17 ■ Triple Heater Channel.

1. Draw a "Chinese clock."* Follow the example below. Include the correspondences for each Element within each segment and color each segment its Five Element color.

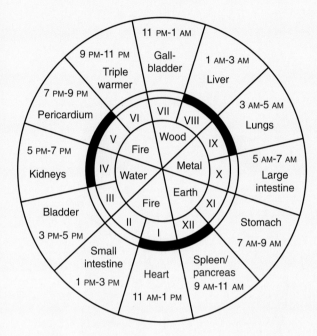

*Figure from Salvo S: *Massage therapy: principles and practice*, ed. 3, St. Louis, 2008, Saunders.

2. Make six copies of the following blank human figure diagrams. On each one, draw a corresponding pair of organ channels, using the color associated with each element. For example, on one diagram draw Stomach and Spleen Channels (Earth element) in yellow, brown, or gold. On another diagram, draw Lung and Large Intestine Channels (Metal element) in a light gray to simulate white. Include key classic tsubo locations.

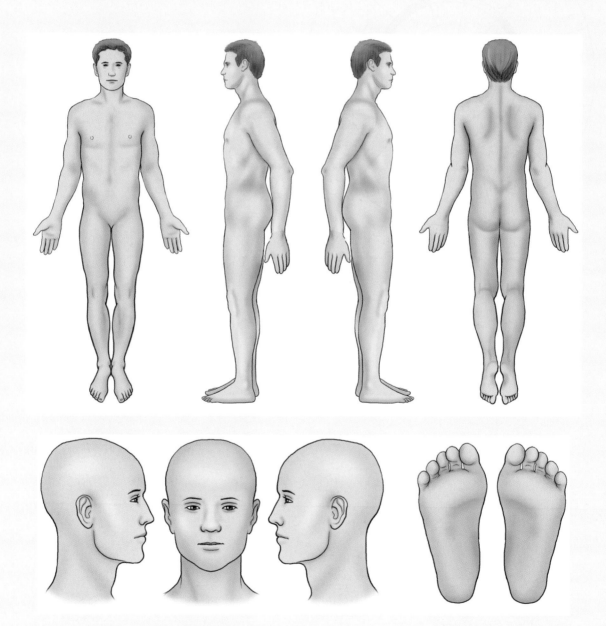

3. Practice palpating channels along their full length and finding tsubo. Do this until you can locate the channels and tsubo without the use of any visual aids, locating them simply by touch.

Notes:

_____

_____

_____

_____

_____

_____

_____

_____

_____

_____

_____

_____

_____

_____

_____

_____

_____

_____

_____

_____

_____

_____

_____

_____

_____

_____

_____

_____

_____

_____

_____

_____

_____

_____

_____

_____

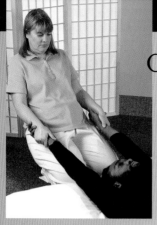

4

SHIATSU CONCEPTS

OBJECTIVES

Upon completion of this chapter, the reader will have the information necessary to do the following:
1. Explain the importance of connection in the shiatsu treatment.
2. Describe ways of achieving focus.
3. Explain Ki connection.
4. Describe the location and importance of the hara.
5. Define the terms kyo and jitsu and give examples of each.
6. Define a tsubo and explain the importance of the tsubo in the shiatsu treatment.
7. Explain the importance of touch sensitivity and intuition in the practice of shiatsu.

Although the history of shiatsu and traditional Asian medical theory provide the foundations for this amazing bodywork, within the actual shiatsu treatment is of course where the melding of theory and practice occurs. The shiatsu treatment itself is where ancient meets contemporary, form meets function, fact meets **intuition**. A strong understanding of the philosophy and concepts behind shiatsu is important. What is more important is that the practitioner be able to translate and use this understanding and have it come through to the client. The primary goal of any shiatsu treatment—or any bodywork treatment, for that matter—is to be with the client in the moment, to work with the client's needs, and to support the client's wellness and healing process.

CONNECTION

The foremost aspect of any shiatsu treatment is the practitioner's **connection** with the client. It is the single most contributory factor to restoring balance and effecting healing change in any therapeutic

Coming from the hara
Completing the Circuit
Connection
Dan Tien
Fixed Tsubo

Focus
Hara
Intuition
Jitsu

Ki Connection
Kyo
Meditation
Mother-hand

Nonfixed Tsubo
Son-hand
Tensegrity
Touch Sensitivity

treatment. Connection is the difference between the practitioner who performs techniques "at" the client's body, and the practitioner who works with the client's mental, physical, emotional, and energetic features. However, connection can be a difficult concept to describe or explain. When it is felt, however, it is the simplest thing in the world.

Connection is that indefinable phenomenon that occurs between living creatures. It can be felt through physical touch as well as energetically and emotionally. Because shiatsu deals with balancing Ki distortions within the client, the practitioner and client need to work in tandem. Harmony between the practitioner and client assists the practitioner in bringing harmony to Ki balance in the client's channels. Some beginning practitioners have the innate ability to connect with and work in harmony with their clients and clients' Ki. Some practitioners need time and experience to develop this skill (Fig. 4-1).

The practitioner needs to have a clear and open mind to be receptive to the client. To assess the client's Ki and restore equilibrium to imbalances in the Ki, shiatsu must be performed with the practitioner in a meditative state. A meditative state means that the practitioner is relaxed, is mentally clear, has put aside personal thoughts not related to the treatment at hand, has released preconceived notions about the client, and is open and ready to be responsive to the information the client gives.

FOCUS

Focus is essential. The beginning practitioner's mind is usually filled with thoughts "Do I have my hands placed correctly?" "Am I on the channel?" "Does this feel **kyo** or **jitsu**?" "What did the client say about when his energy is higher and when it is lower during the day?" These are just a few examples of what could be rushing through the student's mind. Learning how to set thoughts aside and cultivate a meditative state is the first step in the mastery of shiatsu.

As the fletcher whittles and makes straight his arrows, so the master directs his straying thoughts. ~Buddha

There are several ways to do this. One is by practicing traditional **meditation**, which includes stillness of body and stillness of mind (Fig. 4-2).

The relaxed state of awareness that is achieved during meditation is the same relaxed state of awareness that should encompass a shiatsu treatment. Another way is through the practice of moving meditations, such as physical exercise. Regular exercise strengthens the body and nurtures the practitioner's Ki and stimulates its flow and balance. It clears the mind and, provided the exercise is not performed to the limits of the practitioner's endurance, is energizing. The relaxed, clear state felt during exercise is the same state the

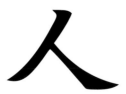

FIGURE 4-1 ■ Kanji for human.

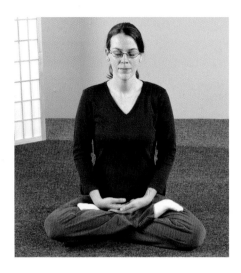

FIGURE 4-2 ■ Traditional meditation.

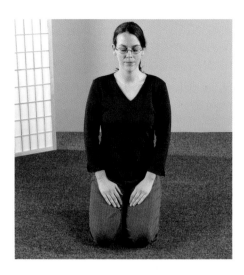

FIGURE 4-3 ■ Seiza.

practitioner should be in while performing shiatsu.

Other examples of moving meditations include Qi Gong (see Chapter 5), martial arts, needlework, gardening, and playing with children and animals. The meditation is not characterized by the actual activity; it is characterized by the calm, unfettered, receptive state of mind the practitioner attains. The practitioner must bring this state of mind into the shiatsu treatment.

If a student is having difficulty achieving an open, clear mind before practicing shiatsu, the following method of centering can be used. It is based on Zen meditation.

Sit comfortably on the floor in seiza. Seiza is a kneeling position in which the gluteals rest on the heels (Fig. 4-3). Rest your hands in your lap. Find a point on the floor approximately 6 feet in front of you, and look at it with an unfocused gaze. Do not close your eyes because that may make you fall asleep. Breathe calmly, and as you breathe in, count "1." As you breathe out, count "2." As you breathe in again, count "3." As you breathe out again, count "4," and so on until you reach 10. Then start over again with counting "1" as you breathe in. If you have thoughts, do not fight them. Let them pass through your mind like birds flying through; do not let them stay and build nests. Breathe this way (counting from 1 to 10, then starting over) for approximately 5 minutes. With practice, you can achieve a centered state that you are able to maintain for the shiatsu treatment.

KI CONNECTION

When the practitioner is centered, relaxed, and has attained an open, receptive mind that is free from distractions, his or her Ki is able to flow freely to connect with the client's Ki. **This Ki connection allows the practitioner to facilitate reharmonizing of Ki imbalances within the client.** The connection is readily transmitted through the practitioner's touch and is palpable to both the practitioner and the client. The tactile techniques that are part of shiatsu are then transformed from simple human-to-human contact to therapeutic treatment.

A feature of Zen shiatsu is two-handed connection on the part of the practitioner. One hand, the **Mother-hand**, remains stationary. It is usually placed nearer to the client's center (his or her belly, or **hara**). The Mother-hand acts as an instrument of baseline measurement of the client's Ki. The practitioner's other hand is the **Son-hand**. It is the hand the practitioner uses to move along the client's channels, assessing the client's Ki by comparing it to the Ki felt by the Mother-hand. The Son-hand is also used to free blockages of Ki, bring Ki to areas that are deficient, and disperse areas that have too much Ki (Fig. 4-4).

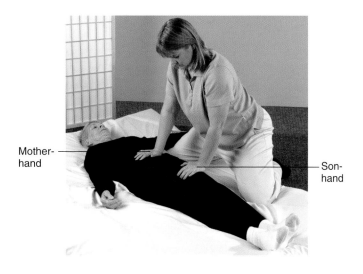

FIGURE 4-4 ■ Mother-hand and Son-hand.

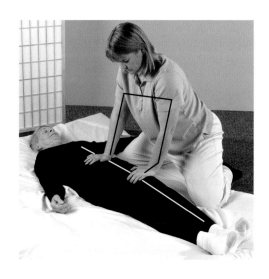

FIGURE 4-5 ■ Completing the circuit of Ki.

The placement of both the practitioner's Mother-hand and Son-hand on the client is known as **completing the circuit** of Ki. The Mother-hand connects with and receives input from the client's Ki. The Ki connection travels through the practitioner, and the practitioner's Ki supports the client's Ki. This reinforced Ki connection travels down through the practitioner's other arm and out through the Son-hand (Fig. 4-5).

HARA

The hara is vital to the practice of shiatsu. It has both physical and energetic components. It is the abdominal area, or the belly, and so it is the core of the body. For those in Asian cultures, it is their center of gravity because traditionally, they spend a great deal of their lives close to the ground, such as sitting on the floor to eat. By contrast, the center of gravity in people of Western cultures is more superior, in the thorax or even the shoulder girdle because most Westerners spend their lives standing or sitting in chairs, not on the ground. A major part of the body mechanics of shiatsu is that the practitioner must "come from his or her hara." In other words, practitioners from Western cultures need to learn to drop their centers of gravity down into their haras, which is necessary for working on futons on the floor. This is discussed further in Chapter 5.

In the center of the hara is the **Dan Tien**, located approximately three fingers' width inferior to the navel. The Dan Tien is the center of the practitioner's Ki, and the practitioner needs to concentrate her Ki coming from this point. The Dan Tien can also be thought of as a pivot point for the practitioner as she moves during the practice of shiatsu (Fig. 4-6).

By focusing breath, Ki, and strength in her hara, the practitioner is able to stay focused and

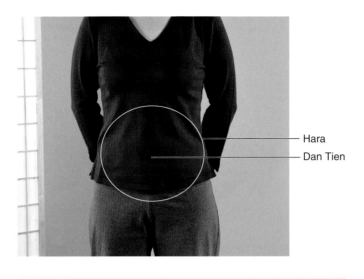

FIGURE 4-6 ■ Hara and Dan Tien.

grounded. **Coming from the hara**, then, is the term used to describe the fusion of relaxed body, centered mind, unrestricted breathing, free flow of Ki, stability, and powerful connection to the Earth (a source of stability and strength) that are essential for the practitioner to perform shiatsu.

The hara is also where Ki can usually be palpated most easily. Some styles of shiatsu incorporate hara assessments (see Chapter 7) as part of the treatment. Although distortions in Ki can occur anywhere in the body, assessing a client's Ki in his or her hara can provide a starting point. Certain channels may manifest as needing treatment more than others and so provide a focus for treatment by the practitioner.

KYO AND JITSU

In shiatsu, treatment plans are designed specifically for each individual client. The plan is based on the client's history from both a traditional Chinese medicine view and a Western medicine view. Five Element Theory can play a role in how the practitioner approaches the session. The client's current physical, emotional, and energetic states, however, provide the most information for the client's immediate needs in the shiatsu session. In other words, the practitioner must be mindful of past issues that can affect the client's well-being as well as present factors.

The shiatsu practitioner can assess the client's needs in the moment in many ways. One is through the questions asked of the client in the pretreatment interview. Another is through visual and auditory assessments of the client. Yet another is energetic assessment done through palpation. All these methods are discussed in more detail in Chapter 7.

Of all the ways to assess a client, palpation of his energetic state is the most direct for the shiatsu practitioner to receive in-the-moment and long-term knowledge. With experience, the practitioner can make the distinction between the two and understand how the two can interact and affect the client. The palpation can be as simple as the practitioner resting her hand on the client with good intention and a clear, receptive mind. As the practitioner performs the treatment, she continually assesses through palpation how to rebalance distortions in the client's Ki.

One particular way for practitioners to work with energetic imbalances involves using the duality that is inherent in the practice of shiatsu. In this case, the duality is represented by the Yin and Yang concepts of full and empty, as in areas of the body that are too full of Ki and areas that are too empty of Ki. This approach is part of Zen shiatsu.

The concept of being full is called *jitsu*. Other meanings of jitsu are excessive and overactive. The concept of being empty" is called *kyo*. Kyo also

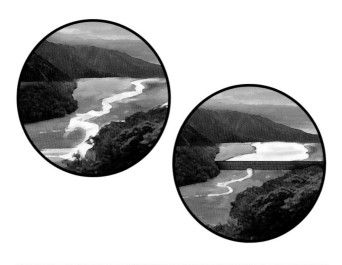

FIGURE 4-7 ■ Kyo and jitsu in flowing and dammed water.

means deficient and underactive. Although they can be viewed as opposing, jitsu and kyo are really two sides of the same coin, the same as Yin and Yang.

Ki can be thought of as flowing through channels much the same way water flows in a stream. If part of the stream becomes blocked or dammed, water no longer flows freely. It will collect in the blocked area (jitsu), and a deficient amount of water will be downstream from the blockage (kyo). When the blockage or dam is removed, water again flows freely (Fig. 4-7).

Just as with the ebb and flow of water, the changing of the seasons, the cycles of weather, and the interconnection of Yin and Yang, jitsu and kyo are inevitable. They are natural, normal responses of the body to changes in the internal and external environment. In some cases the body is able to adapt to changes; sometimes it is not. Sometimes to keep functioning the body will "assign" stress to one particular organ or system. For example, a person's response to stress could be the development of an ulcer (digestive system), headaches (muscular system or cardio-vascular system, depending on whether the headache is muscular or vascular in origin), or insomnia (nervous system). All these disorders can be viewed from Western science perspective, as just described. For example, the headaches could be caused by a possible Liver deficiency (kyo) or excess (jitsu), or the insomnia caused by Heart or Heart Protector being kyo or jitsu.

TENSEGRITY

The relation between kyo and jitsu can best be explained by the **tensegrity** model. Tensegrity is a term coined by architect, engineer, and scientist R. Buckminster Fuller. It is a synthesis of the words "tension" and "structural integrity," and Fuller used this term to describe the revolutionary geodesic domes he designed and constructed, starting in 1949. These domes can sustain their own weight with practically no limits. The basic principle of tensegrity is that, in a stable system, a kind of push-pull relation exists. In the case of geodesic domes, the weight of the building materials is distributed throughout the structure. Weight "pushes" down from the top and is "pulled" through the outwardly curving dome. So if a stress is placed on one part of the system, a change is caused (push) that is compensated for by another part of the system (pull). This ensures the stability of the system. If the compensation does not occur or if the stress is greater than the compensation, the system could break apart (Fig. 4-8).

Jitsu and kyo are examples of tensegrity. If an area of jitsu is present, so will an area of kyo. The integrity of the entire body depends on being able to adapt to changes in Ki flow. Excess Ki in one area causes a rippling effect throughout the entire body; to compensate, Ki will be deficient in another area (Fig. 4-9). Jitsu and kyo can be found in areas as small as a single point on a channel or as large as an entire region of the body. They can

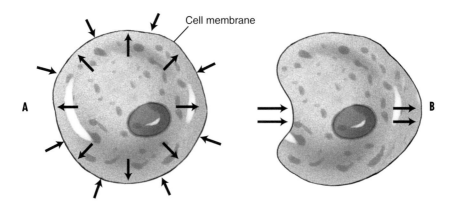

FIGURE 4-8 ■ Tensegrity between a cell and fluid pressures. **A,** Fluid pressure inside the cell pushes outward against the walls of the cell. **B,** Because of the elastic property of the cell membrane, the cell adjusts to the shift in fluid pressure.

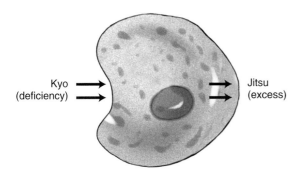

FIGURE 4-9 ■ Cell with kyo and jitsu. Every area of jitsu has a resulting area of kyo. Every area of kyo has a resulting area of jitsu.

TABLE 4-1	Chart of Jitsu and Kyo
Kyo	**Jitsu**
Draws the practitioner in	Pushes the practitioner out
May be less noticeable on palpation	May be more noticeable on palpation
Responds more slowly	Responds more quickly
Feels flaccid	Feels congested, blocked, or dense
May need uninterrupted, penetrating pressure	May need quick, light pressure

manifest in the hara assessment as one channel being the most jitsu and another channel being the most kyo. One part of a channel can be kyo, and another section of the same channel can be jitsu.

Developing the ability to distinguish between jitsu and kyo takes practice. At first, the student practitioner's mind may be so filled with what he is "supposed to be feeling" that he is not able to be clear and centered enough to actually feel. Also of note, kyo and jitsu feel differently to every practitioner; it is a highly personal experience. Each practitioner needs to discover for himself how kyo and jitsu feel to him. Once the practitioner learns this, he is able to connect with jitsu and kyo more and more readily.

Table 4-1 shows a chart that compares jitsu and kyo. It is designed to be a guideline for shiatsu students to follow until they become more comfortable with trusting their intuition.

CLIENT-CENTERED TREATMENT

By being able to distinguish between kyo and jitsu, and understanding sources of issues clients are experiencing, the shiatsu practitioner performs a client-centered treatment specific to the client's needs. Because Ki flows throughout the body in interconnecting channels, any of the push-and-pull distortions of Ki in them, presenting as jitsu and kyo, are expressions of what is happening within the body as a whole. At its simplest, a shiatsu treatment can consist of focusing on the most jitsu channel and the most kyo channel, and by balancing the two any other more minor imbalances will naturally reach equilibrium. In other words, by focusing on the most obviously uneven areas of Ki flow, and evening out these areas, the lesser areas of Ki distortion will be balanced through chain reaction and tensegrity is maintained.

In general, the excess Ki in jitsu areas needs to be dispersed so it can flow to areas of kyo. The deficient Ki in kyo areas needs to be tonified, or supported so that they can gain the needed amount of Ki. Usually kyo areas should be worked first because the more an area is worked, the more Ki is attracted to that area. With various techniques the shiatsu practitioner uses his own Ki to support the client's Ki kyo areas (see Chapter 6); these techniques can also serve to draw excess Ki from jitsu areas. Jitsu areas are worked with techniques designed to diffuse the excess Ki (see Chapter 5).

TSUBO

A *tsubo,* sometimes called a point, is an opening into a channel. It can be a direct link between the channels and the outside world. It has also been described as a gateway because it is a place in which Ki can be changed (dispersed or supported) through thumb or finger pressure or, in the case of acupuncture, through the insertion of a needle. It is represented by the kanji for *jar* (Fig. 4-10).

The jar's widened, bowled bottom represents the channel, and the narrower neck represents the connection of the surface of the body with the channel. While in the kanji the "lid" is

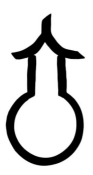

FIGURE 4-10 ■ Kanji for tsubo.

represented as raised and pointed; in reality the opening of the tsubo feels like a small indentation or divot. The thumb or finger should naturally slide into it.

The body has two types of tsubo: fixed and nonfixed. **Fixed tsubo** are the classic tsubo; their locations and effects of addressing them have been studied and recorded for thousands of years. Their locations are set; they are found in virtually the same spot on everyone. The Ki related to the functions of the organs and metabolic processes connect with universal Ki through the fixed tsubo. **Nonfixed tsubo** can occur anywhere along a channel. They reveal the ever-changing Ki flow and manifest as tangible, palpable points that are jitsu or kyo.

Most styles of shiatsu concentrate on the overall flow of Ki through channels. Practitioners assess areas of the body and channels through palpation to determine how evenly the Ki is being distributed and work to even out the flow by unblocking dammed areas and filling deficient areas. Some styles of shiatsu, though, incorporate or even focus on tsubo. They may have prescribed protocols of treatment for particular disorders in which certain tsubo are pressed. Whether or not tsubo are used as the basis of the shiatsu treatment, or are used to supplement the treatment, a knowledge of them can be useful. (See Chapter 3 for classic tsubo descriptions and locations.)

TOUCH SENSITIVITY AND INTUITION

The beauty of shiatsu is in its simplicity. Although a client can present with a variety of symptoms and manifestations, sometimes a simple touch of good intention is enough to balance disharmonies of Ki. Developing **touch sensitivity** starts on the first day of shiatsu (or any bodywork) study and continues throughout the practitioner's lifetime. On occasion great leaps forward occur in palpation skills. Other times advancement happens so incrementally that the student may not be aware of it at all until stopping and reflecting on how much progress she has made.

Along with touch sensitivity is the development of the practitioner's intuition. Touch sensi-

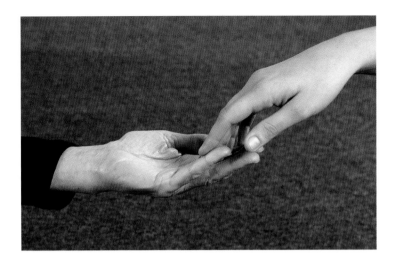

tivity and intuition are the shiatsu practitioner's most powerful tools. They enable the practitioner to determine the best way to work with the client. Although it may seem mysterious to some, everyone has intuition. Sometimes intuition is referred to as having a hunch or gut instinct.

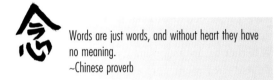

Words are just words, and without heart they have no meaning.
~Chinese proverb

The dictionary defines intuition as "quick and ready insight" and "the power or faculty of attaining direct knowledge or cognition without evident rational thought and inference." The key words are "evident rational thought." In the most uncomplicated explanation, intuition possibly comes from simply piecing together many small bits of information until a complete picture is formed. On the surface it may appear as if no process occurred in how the information about the client's physical and energetic states came together for the practitioner. However, with knowledge and practice the practitioner is able to formulate a "picture" of the client and the client's needs seemingly without effort.

Often the block to intuition is overthinking. If the mind is too busy, it is not receptive to incoming information. Breathing slowly and deeply and emptying the mind allow the practi-

tioner to become receptive. Keeping an awareness in hara gives the practitioner a solid foundation and focus. Sometimes the beginning practitioner may simply need to guess how to best perform the shiatsu treatment. Guessing is the gateway to intuition. A decision has to be made, and the plan and performance of the treatment are based on that decision. With time and experience, the practitioner will no longer guess or "just decide"; he will be genuinely receptive, grounded, open, and intuitive and will be practicing shiatsu accordingly.

Also of note, not every practitioner will be able to work ideally with every client. Many factors can come into play regarding why a practitioner and client are not able to mesh. Beginning shiatsu practitioners need to be aware that, as they are learning and developing their skills, they cannot be the perfect practitioner for every client. Sometimes through clearly definable reasons, or because of inexplicable reasons, the practitioner is not the right fit for a particular client. Practitioners should recognize this possibility and be able to offer referrals of other practitioners to the client.

Many people who are drawn to the field of bodywork do so because of their genuine care and concern for others. They want to help people feel better and help them increase their quality of life. Their compassion makes them exceptionally suitable for the bodywork profession.

However, sometimes bodyworkers easily lose themselves in their work. The line between helping others and taking care of themselves may become blurred. By giving so much of themselves, practitioners can in turn become depleted. Or sometimes clients may make increasing demands on practitioners that practitioners find difficult to refuse.

Practitioners must maintain practitioner-client boundaries. These may be different for each practitioner. However, they should include the idea that clients and practitioners are respectful of each others' time and resources, and neither one should feel taken advantage of by the other.

1. Choose a method of meditation. It could be one you are already doing or one you would like to try. Practice it for 2 weeks and keep a journal of how you feel before, during, and after the meditation. At the end of 2 weeks, take note of changes in the way you feel mentally and physically in the space provided below.

_____

_____

_____

_____

_____

_____

_____

_____

_____

_____

2. Practice palpating kyo and jitsu on recipients. Keep a log of how kyo and jitsu feel in each of the bodies you practice on. Note the commonalities of the kyo areas and the commonalities of the jitsu areas. This can be your guide of how kyo and jitsu feel to you.

_____

_____

_____

_____

_____

_____

_____

_____

_____

_____

3. Write the differences between fixed and nonfixed tsubo.

_____

_____

_____

_____

_____

_____

_____

_____

_____

_____

_____

_____

_____

_____

_____

_____

_____

_____

_____

_____

4. Think of a time in your life when you trusted your intuition. What did it feel like? Were you glad you trusted your intuition? How often do you trust your intuition? How will you use intuition in a shiatsu treatment?

_____

_____

_____

_____

_____

_____

_____

_____

_____

_____

_____

_____

_____

_____

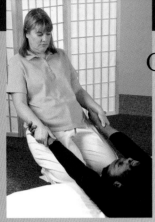

CHAPTER 5

PREPARATION TO PRACTICE SHIATSU

OBJECTIVES

Upon completion of this chapter, the reader will have the information necessary to do the following:
1. Describe the components of the setup for shiatsu.
2. Describe appropriate attire to wear when performing shiatsu.
3. Explain the different components of proper shiatsu body mechanics.
4. Explain self-care methods for the shiatsu practitioner.
5. Perform exercises and stretches that build stamina, increase or maintain flexibility, and increase or maintain balance.
6. Perform each form of Makka-Ho.
7. Explain what Qigong is and perform basic Qigong techniques.
8. Perform each of the basic shiatsu techniques.
9. List the five general principles of treatment.
10. Perform methods of addressing jitsu and kyo.

SHIATSU SETUP

The equipment and setup for shiatsu can be quite different from that of massage therapy. Shiatsu is a relatively simple bodywork treatment, and its setup is relatively simple as well. Shiatsu is usually performed on a futon on the floor. It is covered by a single sheet (Fig. 5-1). Small pillows or bolsters can be used to prop the client comfortably. A scarf can be placed within easy reach for use with certain techniques for the neck (see Chapter 9). Shiatsu can also be performed on a massage table or with the client sitting in a chair.

Soothing music can be played to help the client relax. Hand cleaner, such as witch hazel or diluted alcohol, and a hand towel can also be placed within easy reach. The cleaner can be used to freshen up the client's feet or for the practitioner to clean her hands before working on the client's face.

Key Terms

Body Mechanics	Fire Makka-Ho	Metal Makka-Ho	Three Treasures
Center of Gravity	Hara Headlights	Qigong	Water Makka-Ho
Come from the Hara	Lesser Fire Makka-Ho	Self-Care	Wood Makka-Ho
Earth Makka-Ho	Makka-Ho		

SHIATSU PRACTITIONER CLOTHING

Because of the nature of techniques performed, such as stretches and joint range of motion, both the practitioner and client need to wear comfortable, loose-fitting clothing. Jeans and pants with zippers should not be worn because they inhibit movement and the zippers can pinch the skin during certain shiatsu techniques. Skirts and shorts should not be worn by either the practitioner or client. Because of the movements of the practitioner and the stretches and joint range of

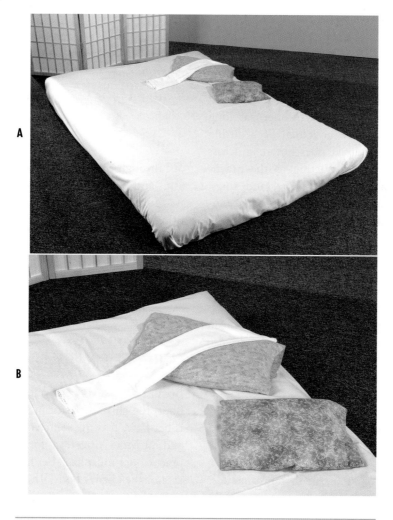

FIGURE 5-1 ■ **A,** Shiatsu setup. **B,** Small pillows with a scarf.

motion the client will experience, skirts and shorts may be too revealing. Additionally, a part of Japanese culture is that there be no skin-to-skin contact between practitioner and client except for the practitioner's hands. While some skin-to-skin contact does occur in the Western practice of shiatsu, pants eliminate much skin-to-skin contact when the practitioner uses his or her knees or legs for support.

The best type of pants to wear is the same as that worn while performing martial arts or any ankle-length pants with either an elastic or drawstring waist. Cotton and cotton-polyester blend (with a high percentage of cotton) are often the most comfortable fabrics for practitioners to wear, but pants made of other fibers, such as linen and hemp, may also be suitable. Scrub pants and sweat pants, as long as they look professional, also suffice. Pants made of fabrics that create obvious sound when moved, such as nylon, should not be worn because the noise can be distracting during the treatment.

Traditionally a long-sleeved shirt would also be worn, but in modern practice a short-sleeved shirt is acceptable. If the practitioner has long hair, he or she should wear it tied back during the treatment to ensure it does not drag across the client or become distracting to the practitioner. Fingernails should be short, and rings, watches, bracelets, dangling necklaces, or dangling (noisy) earrings should not be worn during the treatment. Shiatsu can be done in bare feet as long as the feet are clean or in clean socks (Fig. 5-2).

The practitioner should ask the client to remove his belt, if wearing one, for the treatment so that leg stretches and hip range of motion can be performed more easily. The client should also remove her watch and bracelets and necklaces that may interfere with the treatment.

BODY MECHANICS FOR THE SHIATSU PRACTITIONER

Body mechanics for a massage therapist includes a wide stance supported by flexed knees and a straight back. Strength comes up through the massage therapist's legs, through the torso, then

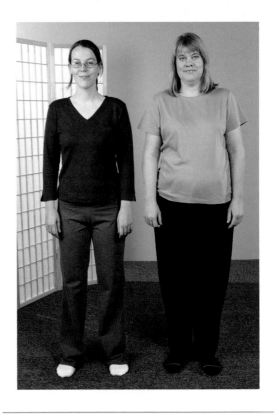

FIGURE 5-2 ■ Appropriate shiatsu apparel.

out through the shoulders and down through the arms and hands (Fig. 5-3).

To be stable and grounded, the shiatsu practitioner needs to have a solid connection with the earth. This is important for steady movement around the client while performing shiatsu techniques. The back must remain straight to prevent straining it while working. This can be thought of as "a connection with the heavens."

CENTER OF GRAVITY

Because shiatsu is performed on a futon on the floor, the shiatsu practitioner's **center of gravity** is her hara. It is the source of her Ki and strength and provides direction for the treatment. The practitioner must keep her hara facing toward the area of the client's body. This helps direct Ki flow from the practitioner to the client and Ki flow within the client. This can be thought of as using **"hara headlights."**

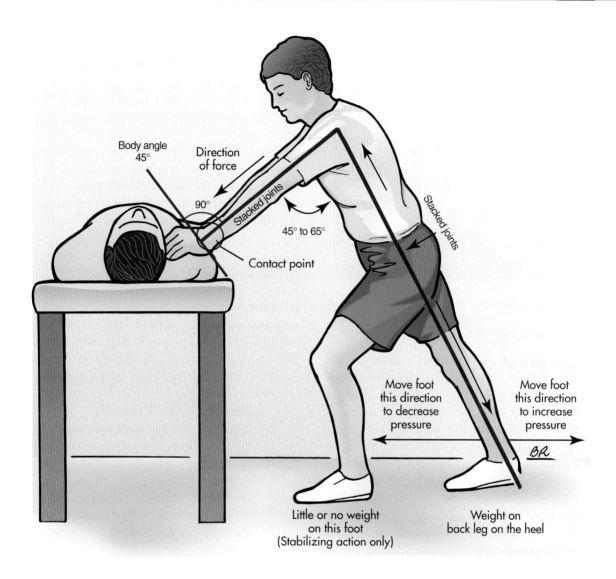

FIGURE 5-3 ■ Massage therapy body mechanics. (From Fritz S: *Mosby's fundamentals of therapeutic massage*, ed 3, St. Louis, 2004, Mosby.)

Because the hara is so significant in the practice of shiatsu, the practitioner should develop her own hara. This can be done by sitting comfortably on the floor, either cross-legged or in seiza. Breath should be focused inward and downward into the hara. Imagining a glow of warmth in the hara can help the expand awareness into the hara. The warmth can then be visualized as extending out through all the channels, muscles, and bones, and out to the fingers, toes, and top of the head. It extends beyond the practitioner's body to connect with the Ki of the universe.

 ## STANCE AND MOVEMENT

To support the hara and give effective treatments, the practitioner must have a stable stance. One way the practitioner can do this is by sitting in a wide seiza position (Fig. 5-4).

A wide seiza is one in which the practitioner's legs are open at least 45 degrees. This position allows smooth pivoting so the practitioner can keep his hara aimed at the area being worked on. To reduce chance of injury to self or the client, the practitioner should never twist or apply techniques at an awkward angle.

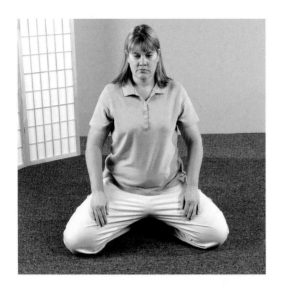

FIGURE 5-4 ■ Shiatsu practitioner in wide seiza.

From this position, the practitioner can rise up to apply more pressure. The strength for application of pressure and Ki connection needs to **come from the hara**, then travel out through the arms and legs. Muscling in from the shoulders or knees can put the practitioner at risk for injury and may hurt the client. The shoulders and arms should be relaxed throughout the treatment.

Other positions a shiatsu practitioner can work from include crawling, squatting, and lunging. Crawling is a movement natural to children and is something that adults generally "forget" how to do. Crawling, however, is a natural way of moving around a client lying on a futon. If necessary, the practitioner can practice crawling until it becomes comfortable again. He should feel his weight shift from hand to hand, knee to knee, and from hands to knees. While crawling, he should use his hara as the center of gravity. Feeling the connection to the earth and the flow of Ki through his body will occur naturally. In time, crawling will be as effortless as walking (Fig. 5-5); also see DVD 5-1.

Squatting is also a natural position for children and is something that adults may need to relearn. Squatting provides a stable base from which to move into other positions easily. Squatting may be difficult at first. The practitioner should practice sinking into a squat and rising from a squat without placing her hands on

the floor for balance. She should use her hara as her center of gravity. Over time her leg muscles will gain strength and balance will improve.

Lunging is modified squatting. Many shiatsu stretches are performed in a lunge position. Reaching certain parts of the client's body is also easier when lunging.

Once comfortable squatting is mastered, movement into a lunge is easy. As with crawling and squatting, the practitioner should use her hara as the center of gravity. Practicing lunging helps build leg strength and improve balance.

THREE TREASURES

In all the positions described previously, as well as seiza and wide-stance seiza, the practitioner must maintain a connection to the earth and a straight back to come from the hara. This can be remembered by using the following "**three treasures**" (Fig. 5-6):

1. **Hara:** the center of the body.
2. **"Point of one hundred meetings":** the top of the head. This point pulls the body upward and keeps the back and posture straight.
3. **"Bubbling spring" (Kidney 1):** the bottom of the foot. This channel keeps the body grounded into the center of the earth.

NECESSITY OF FLUID MOVEMENT

The shiatsu practitioner must incorporate movement into his body mechanics. Flexibility and flow are crucial to smooth, therapeutic treatment, which should be performed as a dance. This may be difficult at first for practitioners who do not have a background in dance. A slight swaying motion can initially be included, then expanded on as he becomes more comfortable with movement and the shiatsu techniques. With experience and practice, dance will naturally become part of the treatment. By practicing the aspects of **self-care**, described in the following section, fluid movement can be developed and enhanced.

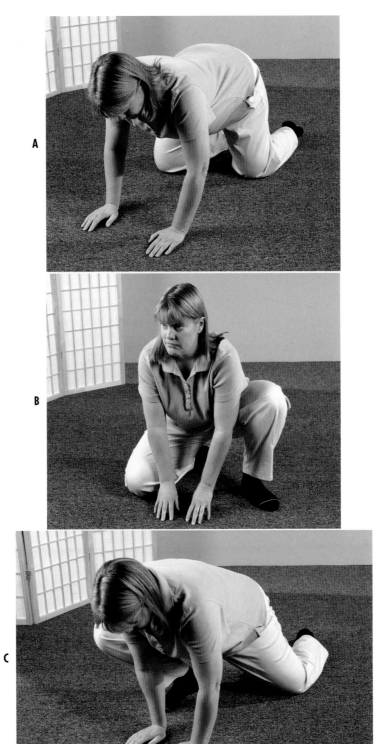

FIGURE 5-5 ■ **A,** Crawling. **B,** Squatting. **C,** Lunging.

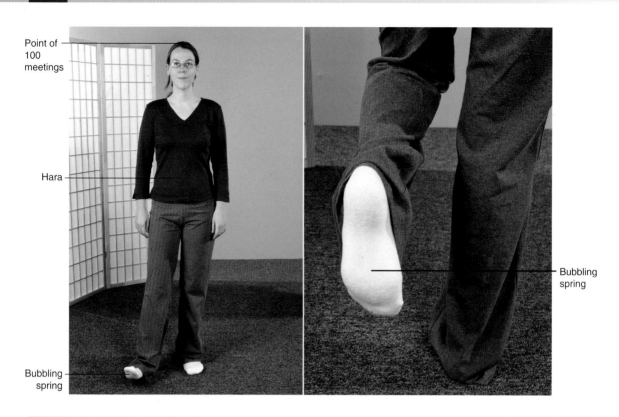

Point of 100 meetings

Hara

Bubbling spring

Bubbling spring

FIGURE 5-6 ■ Two views of the three treasures.

SELF-CARE FOR THE SHIATSU PRACTITIONER

Maintaining health and vitality is critical for the shiatsu practitioner. Aside from the obvious need to avoid sickness and injury, staying healthy ensures that the practitioner has a strong Ki flow, can stay focused, and have the stamina and flexibility necessary to attend to clients' needs.

A good, healthy diet is important. It should be balanced, with emphasis on fruits and vegetables, protein sources, and a high water intake. The foods should be as natural as possible. Overprocessed foods can be low in nutritional value, low in fiber, and high in fat and salt content. The practitioner's diet should help in the work of shiatsu; it needs to provide energy and health and not cause sluggishness (see Chapter 2).

Exercise promotes Ki flow, increases and maintains lung function, increases muscle strength, increases stamina and strength, clears the mind, and increases focus. Exercise can take many different forms: yoga, Pilates, swimming, and walking, to name a few. The point is to do some

sort of movement on a regular basis. It needs to be refreshing and invigorating. How much movement and how often the movement should be done will be different for everyone. The practitioner also needs to spend time focusing inward to clear his mind and take time out from the demands of life. Meditation, whether the traditional sitting meditation, or a moving meditation, such as needlework or gardening, acts as a restorative for body, mind, soul, and Ki.

Renew thyself completely each day; do it again, and again, and forever again.
~Chinese inscription cited by Thoreau in *Walden*

Overexertion and underexertion can also be detrimental to the practitioner's health. If any activity is done to excess Ki is depleted, not enhanced. If the practitioner does not practice movement, Ki flow can slow and become stagnant. Ki can also become stagnant if too much time is spent in stillness, such as too much meditation. This inhibits instead of assists the practitioner in the practice of shiatsu.

BREATHING

Deep, relaxed breathing puts the body in parasympathetic mode and helps the practitioner have clear, focused thought. It also helps to ground the practitioner. She should not have complete awareness of her breathing; the breathing should be so that enough oxygen is being supplied for energy and that she has enough breath to do a treatment smoothly. The practitioner should practice full, deep breathing. The rib cage should expand as she inhales deep into her abdomen. She should then exhale smoothly. Overall, breathing should be done slowly and mindfully. It should not be done too fast or too deeply because of the chance of hyperventilating.

Shiatsu treatments are generally an hour long, so the treatment is fundamentally an hour-long workout. The practitioner must be able to breathe smoothly and evenly throughout the treatment to ensure enough oxygen to do the work. Running out of breath during the treatment or breathing shallowly can be an indication that she is not grounded, or having a stable connection to the earth. The following can be helpful grounding exercises.

EXERCISES AND STRETCHES

To be able to move fluidly during a shiatsu treatment, have stamina, and reduce the risk of injury, the practitioner needs to become flexible (if not already flexible) and maintain that flexibility. Strengthening the body, maintaining or improving balance, and being grounded are also helpful. A series of stretches and exercises can be done to help with flexibility, strength, balance, and being grounded. These can be done as a daily workout or as a warm-up before performing shiatsu treatments. Relax while performing these exercises and stretches, and remember to keep breathing.

 ## FOOT EXERCISES

Flex the toes of both feet and grip them into the floor. Repeat several times (Fig. 5-7, *A*).

While standing on one foot, lift the other foot off the floor in front of you. Circle your foot clockwise several times, then counterclockwise several times. Repeat with your other foot (Fig. 5-7, *B*).

While standing on one foot, lift the other foot off the floor in front. Plantarflex then dorsiflex your ankle several times. Repeat with the other foot (Fig. 5-7, *C*).

 ## LEG AND HIP EXERCISES

While keeping your back straight, sink into a squat and hold for several seconds. Rise up again and sink back into a squat. Repeat several times (Fig. 5-8, *A*).

While keeping your back straight, sink into a squat, lunge to one side and hold for several seconds, then release. Come back to the center, lunge to the other side and hold for several seconds, then release. Repeat from side to side several times (Fig. 5-8, *B*).

Turn to face one side. Bring one leg forward and move the other leg backward. Place both hands on the floor next the medial side of the foot of the forward leg. While keeping your back straight, lunge forward and hold for several seconds, then release. Turn to the other side and repeat (Fig. 5-8, *C*).

Sit on the floor with both legs stretched out in front of you. Flex one knee and grasp your foot with both hands. While holding your foot at stomach level and keeping your back straight, pull your foot forward. The stretch should be felt in your gluteal muscles. Hold for several seconds, then release. Lay your leg back down on the floor and repeat the stretch with your other leg (Fig. 5-8, *D*).

 ## BACK STRETCH

While lying flat on the floor, flex both hips and grasp behind your knees with both hands. While keeping your back on the floor, pull your knees toward your chest. The stretch should be felt in your back. Hold for several seconds, then release (Fig. 5-9).

 ## NECK STRETCHES

Flex your neck forward. Interlace your fingers and place them on the back of your head. Pull

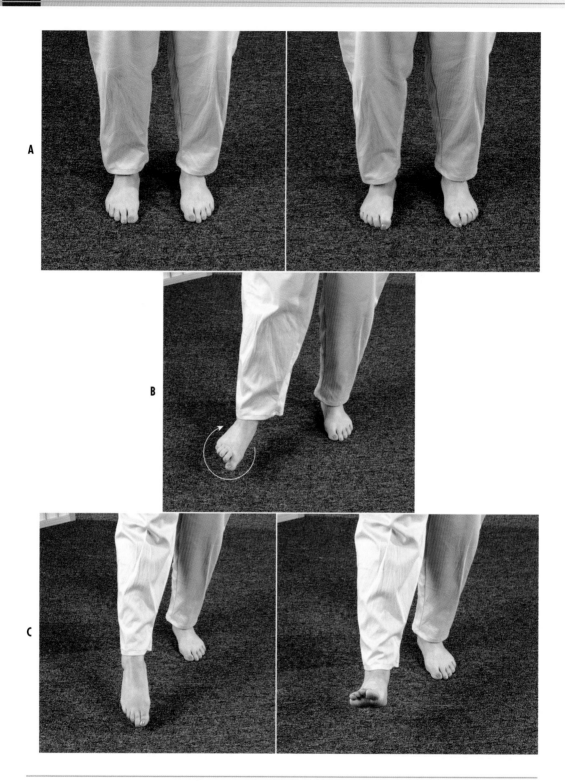

FIGURE 5-7 ■ **A,** Toe grips. **B,** Ankle circles. **C,** Plantarflexion and dorsiflexion.

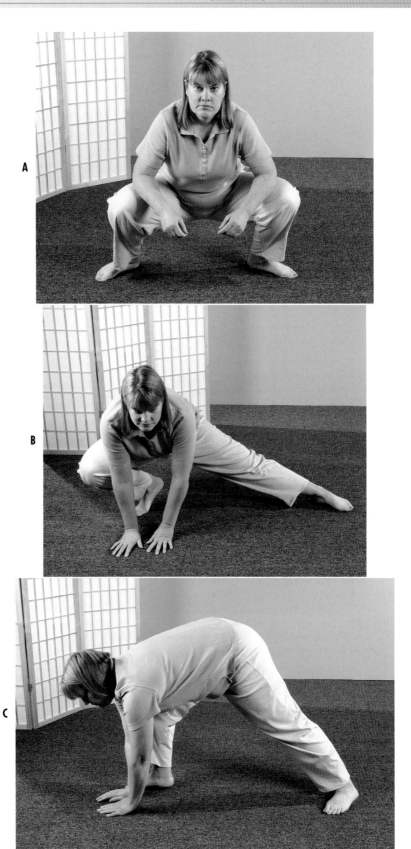

FIGURE 5-8 ■ **A,** Standing squat. **B,** Squat with lateral lunge. **C,** Forward lunge.

Continued

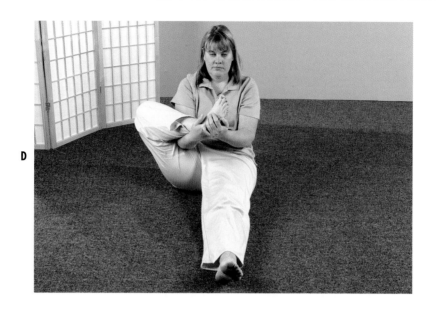

FIGURE 5-8, cont'd ■ **D,** Sitting gluteal stretch.

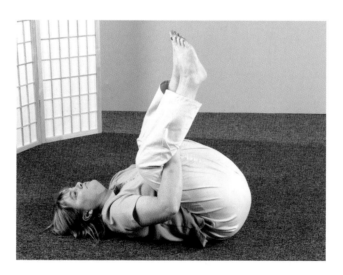

FIGURE 5-9 ■ Back stretch.

your head down gently for a posterior neck stretch. Hold for several seconds, then release (Fig. 5-10, *A*).

Flex your neck backward until your face is toward the ceiling. Gently stretch your anterior neck for several seconds, then release (Fig. 5-10, *B*).

Laterally flex your neck. Place your hand from the same side on top of your head and gently stretch your neck. Hold for several seconds, then release. Bring your head to center, then laterally flex your neck to the other side and repeat (Fig. 5-10, *C*).

5-6 ARM AND SHOULDER EXERCISES

Extend one arm out in front, just below shoulder height. With your other hand, grasp the fingers of the hand on the extended arm. Pull the hand into extension. The stretch should be felt in your an-terior forearm. Hold for several seconds, then release. Repeat with your other arm (Fig. 5-11, *A*).

Horizontally abduct both arms, at approximately shoulder height. Continue abducting

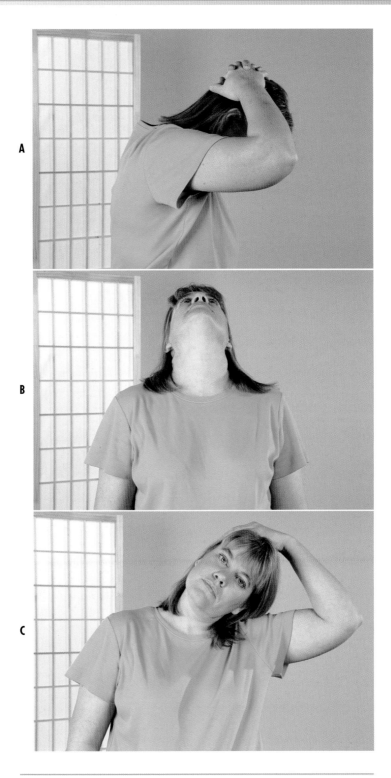

FIGURE 5-10 ■ **A,** Posterior neck stretch. **B,** Anterior neck stretch. **C,** Lateral neck stretch.

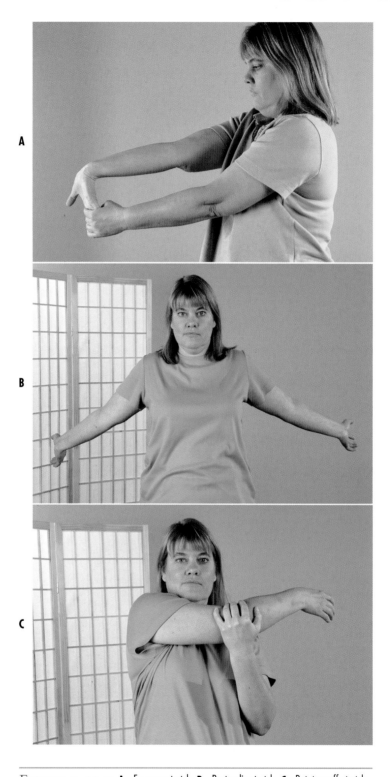

FIGURE 5-11 ■ **A,** Forearm stretch. **B,** Pectoralis stretch. **C,** Rotator cuff stretch.

your arms horizontally until you feel a stretch in pectoralis major. Hold for several seconds, then release (Fig. 5-11, *B*).

With your elbow extended, horizontally adduct one arm across your body at shoulder height. Place your other hand on your extended elbow and push your arm gently toward your chest until a stretch is felt in the rotator cuff muscles. Hold for several seconds, then release. Repeat with the other arm (Fig. 5-11, *C*).

 ## HAND EXERCISES

Grasp each finger of one hand with the thumb and forefinger of the other hand. Gently perform joint range of motion clockwise several times, then counterclockwise several times. Repeat with the fingers of the other hand (Fig. 5-12, *A*).

Place your fingertips together in a tentlike position. Gently push your hands together until you feel a stretch in your fingers. Hold for several seconds, then release (Fig. 5-12, *B*).

Interlace your fingers together in front of you. Pronate your forearms so that your palms are facing down. Extend your elbows and push your fingers into a gentle stretch. Hold for several seconds, then release (Fig. 5-12, *C*).

From a standing position and while keeping your back straight, flex your knees and place your fingertips on the floor. Lean forward and rest your weight on your fingertips. Over time, this will strengthen your fingers (Fig. 5-12, *D*).

 ## EXERCISE TO IMPROVE BALANCE

Stand with your feet shoulder-width apart. Flex one knee so that the sole of the foot is facing the hamstrings. While balancing on the other foot, grasp the elevated foot with the hand on the same side and pull it as close to your hamstrings as possible. Extend the arm on the other side over your head. Hold this position for several seconds as your body settles into a stable balance. Release, then repeat with the foot on the other side (Fig. 5-13).

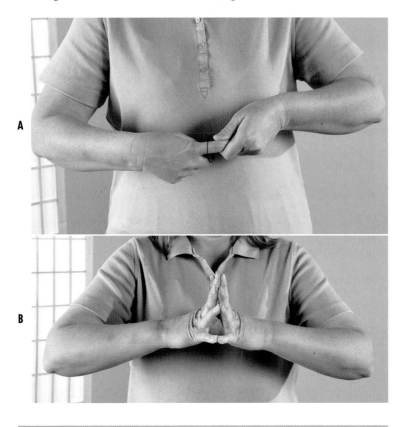

FIGURE 5-12 ■ **A,** Range of motion of each finger. **B,** Finger stretch.   *Continued*

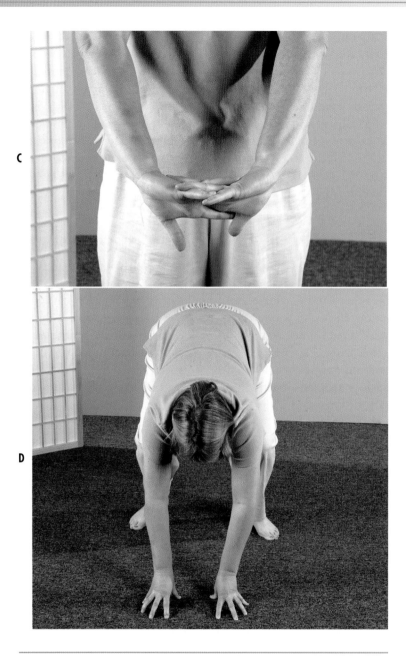

FIGURE 5-12, cont'd ▪ **C,** Finger stretch. **D,** Leaning weight on fingers to strengthen them.

5-9 MAKKA-HO

In the 1970s a Japanese man named Makka designed a series of stretches based on the channel pairs. These are known as **Makka-Ho,** which means Makka's method, or Makka's exercises. This routine of stretches provides several benefits. They serve as a reminder for channel locations; they provide an overall stretch because every area of the body is addressed; and they can bring to the shiatsu practitioner awareness of imbalances in his own body. If tension, tightness, or pain is felt while performing the Makka-Ho for a particular set of channels, there may be jitsu or kyo issues in those channels. As with all exercises and

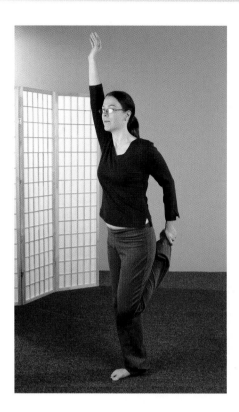

FIGURE 5-13 ■ Exercise to improve balance.

stretches, it is important to relax while doing them and to remember to keep breathing.

METAL MAKKA-HO

Stand with your feet shoulder-width apart. Behind your back, form an interlocking circle with the thumb and middle finger of both hands. Point your index fingers. While inhaling, lean back. Hold for several seconds. Release, and lean forward while exhaling, flexing your trunk so that your back is parallel to the floor. Hold for several seconds, release, and stand upright. Interlock your other thumb and middle fingers behind your back again and repeat the Makka-Ho (Fig. 5-14, A-C).

EARTH MAKKA-HO

Earth Makka-Ho can be done several ways. One is the same method described in the exercise to improve balance. Stand with your feet shoulder-width apart. Flex one knee so that the sole of the foot is facing the hamstrings. While balancing on the other foot, grasp the elevated foot with the hand on the same side and pull it as close to your hamstrings as you can. Extend the arm on the

other side over your head. Hold this position for several seconds as you feel your body settle into a stable balance. Release, then repeat with the foot on the other side (Fig. 5-14, D).

Another method is to sit in on the floor in seiza. Move your feet outward so they are just lateral to your gluteals. Lie down with your back flat on the floor. Raise both arms over your head and lay them flat on the floor. Hold for several seconds, then release (see Fig. 5-14, D).

A third way is a modified version of the above method. Lie with one foot close to your gluteals and the other leg stretched out straight on the floor. Raise both arms over your head and lay them flat on the floor. Hold for several seconds, then release. Repeat with the leg that was stretched out flat now tucked close to the gluteals, and the leg with the knee that was flexed now stretched out straight (see Fig. 5-14, D).

WATER MAKKA-HO

Sit on the floor with your legs stretched out straight in front of you. Raise both your arms straight over your head. While keeping your back and arms straight, flex your trunk and bring your hands toward your feet. See if you can touch KI 1 (bubbling spring) with your fingers. Hold for several seconds, then release (Fig. 5-14, E and F).

FIRE MAKKA-HO

Sit on the floor with your knees flexed and the soles of your feet placed against each other. Interlace your fingers and grasp your feet with them. Pull your feet as close into your body as is comfortable, and let your knees relax as much as possible. Inhale, and while keeping your back straight, flex your trunk and lean forward as far as you can while exhaling, keeping your elbows outside your knees. Breathe as you hold this position for several seconds, then release (Fig. 5-14, G).

LESSER FIRE MAKKA-HO

Sit on the floor with your legs crossed. Tuck your inside foot close to your body. Cross your arms and place your hands in front of your knees. Inhale. As you exhale, flex your trunk to lean forward as far as possible, elongating your arms on the floor as much as is comfortable. Breathe as you hold this position for several seconds, then release (Fig. 5-14, H).

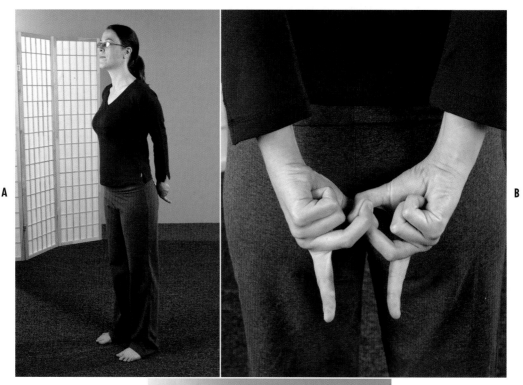

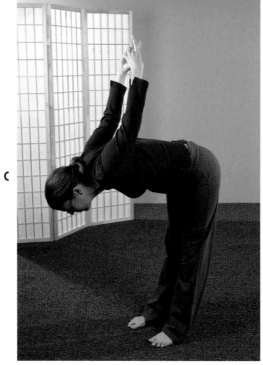

FIGURE 5-14 ■ **A-C,** Metal Makka-Ho.

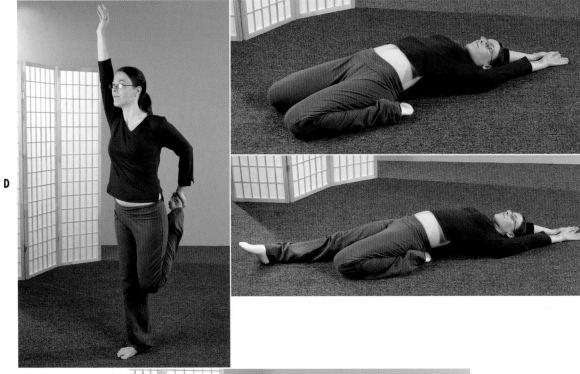

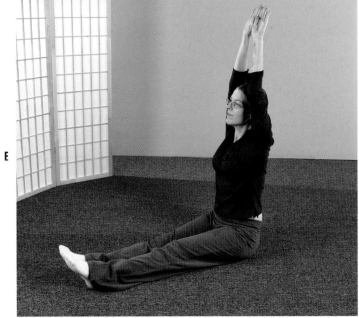

FIGURE 5-14, cont'd ■ **D,** Earth Makka-Ho. **E,** Water Makka-Ho.

Continued

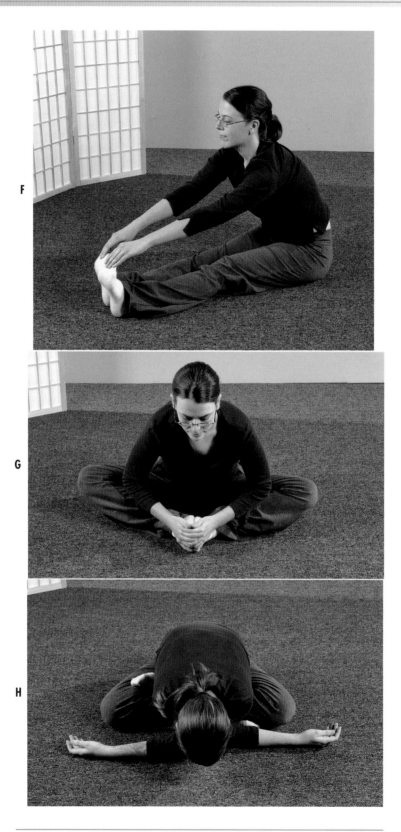

FIGURE 5-14, cont'd ■ **F,** Water Makka-Ho. **G,** Fire Makka-Ho. **H,** Lesser Fire Makka-Ho.

WOOD MAKKA-HO

Sit on the floor with your legs stretched out straight at a 45-degree angle from your body. Raise one arm over your heard and keep it extended. While keeping your back straight, laterally flex to the opposite side as the raised arm. Extend the arm on this side toward your foot. Hold for several seconds, then release and come to center. Laterally flex to the other side and repeat. After releasing, come to center. While keeping your back straight, flex your trunk and, as you lean forward, stretch your arms straight out in front of you as far as you can. Hold for several seconds, then release (Fig. 5-15).

QIGONG*

The ancient practice of **Qigong** is performed specifically to help the practitioner focus on developing Ki, breath, and awareness. It increases flexibility and stamina, improves strength, and is a form of moving meditation. In fact, by practicing this one type of movement, the shiatsu practitioner can accomplish most of what is necessary to maintain health.

WHAT IS QIGONG?

Qigong (also known as Chi Gong or Chi Kung) originated in China many thousands of years ago. As mentioned in Chapters 1 and 2, *Qi* can be translated as breath or energy (and in this text is generally used noted its Japanese form, *Ki*. However, because Qigong is a Chinese practice, *Qi* will be used instead of *Ki* in this discussion of Qigong.). The breath referred to is not simply the air taken into and out of the lungs; it also includes, perhaps more appropriately, the more subtle breath or energy in the body. Bioelectric energy is the energy of the body and of all living creatures. In a larger view, Qi is the energy or force that keeps things coherent—from the subatomic particles that make up atoms to the force that pervades the cosmos. *Gong* translates as practice or cultivation. You may gong, or cultivate, many things from gardening, honing musical ability, or continuing your practice of bodywork. You may therefore think of Qigong as cultivating the subtle

*Contributed by Bob Lehnberg.

energy of your body and its relationship to others and to your environment. The practice of Qigong is an activity, and Qi itself is a tangible, felt quality in the body. People of any age can practice Qigong.

Qigong is practiced for many reasons. Some of these reasons include improving health and longevity, attaining spiritual enlightenment, increasing internal energy to develop power (as in martial arts), and developing the ability to help others heal themselves through Qi connection. In this chapter, Qigong is discussed to improve personal health and alignment, thereby increasing effectiveness when working with clients. The clearer and stronger your Qi, the more likely you are to be efficient in your treatments because less effort will be necessary to connect with your client's Qi. You are also less likely to take on your clients' energy patterns or issues because your will be more strongly centered in yourself.

The health benefits of Qigong are many. They include improving balance, strengthening the legs, releasing the lower back, aligning the spine, improving body mechanics, improving internal organ function, increasing immunity, calming and centering the mind, increasing and organizing energetic reservoirs and pathways, becoming present, and releasing aberrant energetic configurations of the past. Overall, practicing Qigong enhances consciousness of body, mind, and spirit while instilling an appreciation of relationship and connection with others, nature, and the universe.

ENERGY ORGANIZATION OF THE BODY

A person's well of energy resides in the belly a few inches below the navel and halfway back to the spine, in the center of the gut. This location is referred to as the *dan tien,* which translates to "sea of Qi" or "elixir field," among other names. It is a reservoir of energy akin to a reservoir of water that serves the needs of the surrounding community.

The dan tien connects to a system of deep conduits through which energy can flow. Traditional Chinese medicine refers to these as the "Eight Extraordinary Vessels" or the "Eight Strange Flows." Only three of these are considered in this text, with the addition of one more (four in total). For information on the other vessels, consult a text of traditional Chinese medicine.

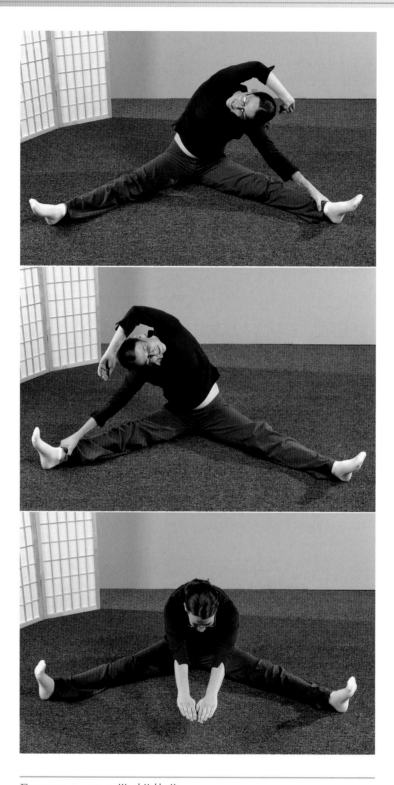

FIGURE 5-15 ■ Wood Makka-Ho.

The Central Channel ("Thrusting Channel") is the central energetic axis and runs from *hui yin* ("point of most Yin," or "earth's gate"), located in the perineum between the anus and the genitals, to *bai hui* ("meeting of one hundred points") located at the crown of the head. This point is akin to the *shushumna nadi* in yoga terminology.

The Governing Vessel runs up the midline of the body from hui yin back through the coccyx; up through the sacrum, spine, and neck; around the head; through bai hui; and down the forehead to the palate behind the upper teeth. From here, the tongue connects this point of the Governing Vessel to the Conception Vessel, which runs down the midline of the body through the tongue; down the front of the neck, sternum, abdomen, and pubic disc; and ends at hui yin. Diagrams of the locations of the Governing Vessel and Conception Vessel as well as discussions of them are in the Appendix.

The Belt Vessel ("Girdle Vessel") runs horizontally around the body through the dan tien (a few inches below the navel) in front and *ming men* ("the gate of life") in back. Ming men is located between the third and fourth lumbar vertebrae. Because the dan tien is a bit lower than ming men, the Belt Channel does not run perfectly in the horizontal plane. It connects the vertically running channels of energy.

A system of smaller pathways connects with the extraordinary vessels and forms the 14 organ channels (the 12 organ channels discussed in Chapter 3, plus the Governing Vessel and Conception Vessel). These are the most commonly used channels by practitioners of acupuncture, acupressure, and shiatsu. Some forms of Qigong have been developed specifically to cultivate the organ channels. These forms are more intricate than will be considered in this text.

The energy system of the dan tien, vessels, and channels is interconnected; as a person becomes nourished and filled, this energy flows over to the other linked systems. For example, as energy is increased in the dan tien, the excess flows over into the channels. When they are full, the organ channels are filled. Conversely, as the channels get full, the excess energy spills over into the vessels, which then feed into the dan tien.

The select Qigong forms presented in this text nourish the dan tien and the larger vessels, which will then encourage quality and quantity of flow in the organ channels. In this way, Qigong practice, along with giving and receiving shiatsu treatments, work together to increase energy reserves and circulation.

PREPARING TO PRACTICE QIGONG

A practice session involves three main actions: warming up, the Qigong practice itself, and closing. While all three actions do not always need to be done, the greatest benefit may be found by following this sequence. When time and circumstances are not ideal, doing any part is better than doing none at all.

Practicing outside is best because the air quality is generally fresher and the Qi more abundant, though weather and urban conditions sometimes prevent this. Practicing in the wind, rain, or extreme cold is not beneficial. Excessive noise or odor also tend to disturb the Qi.

You may want to practice in the morning, after a shower and a bowel movement and before eating breakfast; a small snack may ease hunger pangs. If morning is not convenient, any time is better than not at all, though waiting at least 2 hours after eating a meal is best.

Walks

You may want to begin your practice with a regular stroll or start with one of the walks described below. Walking stirs movement of the blood and the Qi and helps you begin the practice. The very nature of walking entails a complete weight shift from one side to the other to ensure a fuller differentiation and integration of Yin (weight-bearing side) and Yang (mobile side).

These walks can be done at a slow or fast pace. Ideally these walks are done outdoors, but if they must take place in an indoor space, they can be done at a slower pace. Following are two of many walks to practice:

- The "puppet walk" has many similar qualities of movement to a marionette puppet. Begin standing as though your head is suspended by a string from the heavens. Rest your left hand at your side and your right hand, palm facing inward, in line with your right thigh and knee. Energetically connect the palm of your hand to the knee. Inhale and lift the hand and knee simultaneously so that the distance between the palm and the knee remains the same. The movement of the palm initiates the movement of the knee through the energetic connection. Raise the hand and knee until the thigh is parallel to the floor. The palm will be parallel to the floor. Exhale and lower the palm and knee down until the heel touches the floor. Then roll your weight onto this foot, which fully receives the weight of the whole body. The left side is now empty of weight and the left hand floats up in line with your left thigh with the palm over the knee. On the inhale, continue to lift the palm, which initiates the lifting of the knee. Throughout the puppet walk, maintain a vertical spine and do not let your head lower or bob when you raise the hand and leg.

■ The "Belt Vessel walk" entails a casual walking stride while you trace, energetically massage, and balance the Belt Vessel. With your arms down at your sides, create space in your armpits and round your arms and hands as though mimicking a hoop skirt. As you walk, swing your arms and hands back on the inhale and energetically connect your palms and ming men. Swing your hands forward on the exhale and energetically connect your palms with the dan tien. Relax as you trace the belt channel and connect the dan tien and ming men with your palms as they slowly swing forward and back in rhythm with the breath. This movement does not need to be coordinated with the gait of your legs, though you may find a natural coordination and rhythm. Remember to relax and maintain a vertical spine.

Breathing

Breathing is the essence of Qigong. External respiration occurs when air goes in and out of the lungs on inhalation and exhalation. Internal respiration, which may be referred to as the energetic

breath, occurs at the cellular level; oxygen moves from the blood into the cell and carbon dioxide moves from the cell into the blood. The subtlest level of respiration is the use of oxygen within the cell to generate energy and the formation of carbon dioxide as a waste product.

In normal abdominal breathing the belly moves out, away from the spine, on the inhale; the belly moves in toward the spine on the exhale. After you practice this rhythm and it becomes natural, add the energetic breath. The energetic breath is attained through a pause or suspension of the breath at the end of the inhalation and the end of the exhalation. The pause is maintained through the muscles and tissues of the trunk and can last from a moment to many seconds depending on the clarity and health of your system. Note that breath suspension does not occur through the closure of the vocal diaphragm; the throat and neck remain soft and relaxed the entire time. The importance of eventually adding the energetic breath to Qigong practice cannot be overemphasized. With practice, breath suspension can be held for longer periods of time with no effort or discomfort.

The sequence may be practiced as follows:
1. Inhale and gather air as the lungs expand.
2. Suspend the inhalation breath and allow the tissues of the entire body to expand.
3. Exhale and release air as the lungs condense.
4. Suspend the exhalation breath and allow the tissues of the entire body to condense.
5. Repeat.

WARMUPS

Warming up gently gets the blood moving, warms connective tissues, and generally helps loosen the tissues of the body. It also helps move the consciousness from the head into the body. As you warm up, breathe naturally, relax, and move in a comfortable way. Each time you warm up, choose a different order of the following activities depending on your state of mind, restfulness, and overall sense of well-being.

Stand comfortably with feet parallel to each other and approximately shoulder width apart. Place your hands at your sides.

- **Hand shaking:** Lift your hands in front of your body with forearms parallel to the earth. Shake your hands (rapidly pronate and supinate); allow your thumb to move freely.

- **Wrist rotations:** Gently extend your fingers and slowly rotate your hands at the wrists. Do this in both directions.

- **Body bouncing:** While facing forward, gently and fluidly bounce your entire body, allowing the movement to come from the feet. Relax and let all the tissues of the body become involved in the movement.

- **Side-to-side body swings ("knocking on the gate of life"):** Place your feet slightly wider than shoulder width apart and gently rotate your body side to side, with your arms relaxed and suspended from the shoulder joints like pendulums. Rotate your torso side to side and let your hands swing freely. In a relaxed way, bend your elbows just enough to bring your hands in contact with the ming men (middle lumbar area) when swinging to the back and the dan tien (just below the navel) when swinging to the front. The contact of your hands with your body is a gentle patting rather than a forceful striking.

- **Shoulder girdle rotations:** Center yourself then slowly rotate your shoulder girdle in the forward direction; shift your shoulder girdle forward, upward, backward, downward, and then forward again. Repeat 10 times. Do this in the reverse direction; shift your shoulder girdle backward, downward, forward, upward, and then backward again. Repeat 10 times. During shoulder girdle rotations, be sure to keep your arms and shoulder joints relaxed. Move slowly enough to feel your tissues moving.

- **Arm rotations:** Rotate your arms in full circles from the shoulder joints; your shoulder girdles should also move. Make full rotations to the front as though swimming the butterfly stroke. Repeat this in the reverse direction. Now swing your arms in opposite directions, with one arm rotating forward and the other rotating in the reverse direction. Switch directions. When doing these grand arm rotations, extreme movements are not necessary because your ease and comfort are more important than range.

- **Head and neck rotations:** Move your head forward and rotate it to the right by bringing the right ear toward the right shoulder. Pause and release the head forward to midline, then rotate it to the left by bringing the left ear toward the left shoulder. Pause and repeat to the right. By only going in a half circle to the front, you avoid straining the joints of the cervical vertebrae. Do this movement slowly enough to feel your tissues moving.

- **Waist rotations:** Place your hands on your pelvis for stabilization and rotate your head, torso, and waist in a counterclockwise direction (forward, left, back, right, forward, and continue). The crown of your head makes a circle in space while your pelvis and legs remain still and stable. You may make small or large circles depending on your preference and state of fitness. Repeat rotations in the reverse direction.

- **Pelvis rotations:** Place your hands on your pelvis. Rotate your pelvis in a counterclockwise direction. The crown of your head is still while everything below (neck, torso, pelvis, and legs) rotates. Maintain your pelvis in neutral position and keep it facing forward through the entire range of rotation. You may make small or large circles depending on your preference and state of fitness. Repeat rotations in the reverse direction. These moves can also be done while sitting down.

- **Knee rotations:** Place your feet together. Flex your knees and hips and place your hands on your knees. Make small counterclockwise circles with your knees. You should initiate movement at the ming men (approximately the middle of the lumbar spine) while the rest of your body, including your knees, follows along. This is different than initiating movement in your knees and possibly placing more stress on them than needed. Also, to begin with, do not let your knees move too far in front of your toes. You may increase your range of rotation with practice.

- **Ankle rotations:** Shift your body weight to one foot and place the tips of the toes of the other foot on the floor. The toes should have minimal pressure on the floor. Rotate your ankle joint as the heel makes circles and your toes pivot on the floor. Repeat in the reverse direction. Repeat with the other side. Wearing shoes can make this movement more comfortable on your toes.

QIGONG PRACTICE

Standing

Standing is arguably the most important Qigong practice. Even though the position requires no external movement, the mind and Qi are moving within the stillness of the body. Below are two forms of standing; the basic stance and the horse stance. The basic stance is physically easier than the horse stance.

When beginning standing practice, start with only a few minutes. If you stand for too long at first and exhaust yourself, you may become disenchanted with standing and forego this part of your practice. As you develop strength and endurance, gradually increase your standing time to 20 minutes. During each standing session, resist the urge to move or fidget. Moving and fidgeting are positive signs that your body is clearing old, errant energy patterns. Clear your mind and continue to breathe in an effortless manner.

Relaxation is a key to standing and moving Qigong. This does not mean being limp. Relaxation is more appropriately considered as using the least amount of energy or tension needed to accomplish a particular stance or movement form. The Chinese term for this is *sung*. When relaxing in a standing position or form, keep the concept of sung in mind.

Within each stance are many nuances of alignments. Described below are some of the basic alignments.

Key alignments of the basic stance are as follows (Fig. 5-16):

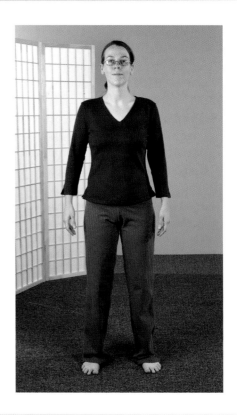

FIGURE 5-16 ■ Basic stance.

- Place feet shoulder width apart and parallel to each other.
- Slightly bend knees to a position not forward of the mid-foot.
- Slightly fold (flex) hip region.
- Slightly round the spine from head to tail.
- Release (drop) the tail toward a spot between the arches of the feet.
- Effortlessly lift the head as though suspended by a cord from the heavens.
- Release chin slightly down and back while leaving the throat open.
- Connect the tip of the tongue to the upper palate, behind the upper teeth.
- Spread the arms to open a small space in the armpit area.
- Turn the palms of the hands to face the thighs.
- Align the middle finger with the lateral thigh (along the pants seam).
- Relax the entire body.

The horse stance is more challenging and more readily cultivates strength in the legs and

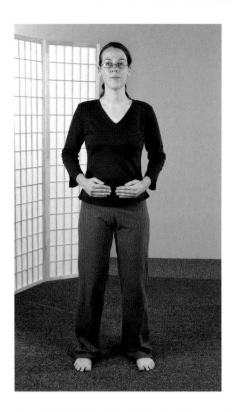

FIGURE 5-17 ■ Horse stance.

arms while developing greater power in the dan tien.

Key alignments of the horse stance are as follows (Fig. 5-17):

- Place feet twice shoulder width apart and parallel to each other.
- Bend knees as much as comfortably possible while maintaining them behind the toes; align knees over the second toe.
- Bend hips as though preparing to sit down in a chair.
- Slightly round spine from head to tail.
- Release (drop) the tail toward a spot between the arches of the feet.
- Effortlessly lift the head as though suspended by a cord from the heavens.
- Release chin slightly down and back while leaving the throat open.
- Connect the tip of the tongue to the upper palate, behind the upper teeth.
- Raise hands in front to chest level and round arms as though hugging a tree.

- Turn the palms to face the dan tien, with the fingers of each hand pointing toward each other.
- Relax the shoulders and lower the elbows below the wrists.
- Relax the entire body.

Feeling Qi

To feel Qi between your hands, begin in the basic stance. Relax, bend your elbows, and bring your palms up until your forearms are parallel with the earth. Rub your hands together until you feel the warmth. On an inhalation, allow your hands to move apart. On the exhalation, allow them to move toward each other. Continue until an expanding feeling occurs between your hands (particularly the palms) on the inhalation and a contracting feeling on the exhalation. You may feel a pull or a push between your palms as you move them together and apart in sync with your breathing rhythm. This is the sensation of Qi of the body.

Pulsing the Three Dan Tiens

The following set of movements engages the opening and closing of the three dan tiens of the body. Pulsing refers to repetitions of closing and opening the body centers as the body sinks and rises. The lower dan tien, as previously discussed, is located slightly below the navel and deep in the belly. The middle dan tien is located in the center of the chest, and the upper dan tien is located between the eyebrows and is also known as the "third eye." First pulse the lower dan tien, then the middle dan tien, then the upper dan tien. You can begin with nine repetitions of pulsing each dan tien. With time, you can increase the number of repetitions.

Start in the basic stance. Bend your elbows and bring your hands in front of the lower dan tien in a relaxed circle. Turn your palms to face your belly. The fingertips of each hand are a few inches apart and point toward one another. Relax your hands and lower your thumbs. Relax your shoulders and entire body. Exhale, shift your weight onto your heels and close the lower dan tien by bringing your palms closer to your belly. Sink your entire body as you bend your knees and hips (as though you were going to sit in a chair) and slightly curve your spine. Inhale, press K1 into the earth, and open the lower dan tien by moving your palms move away from your belly. Your arms open out horizontally and your hands do not rise during this opening. Raise your entire body as you extend your legs and spine. End with your spine vertical and your arms and hands open as though embracing a large tree. Continue this sequence of closing and opening the body nine times. With time and practice you may feel the Qi collect at the dan tien as you bring the hands in and radiate as you open the hands out (Fig. 5-18).

At the end of the ninth opening, raise your hands to chest level. Repeat the movements of closing and opening as above except now you are pulsing the middle dan tien. Keep your shoulders relaxed and your elbows lower than your wrists. Open and close nine times (Fig. 5-19).

At the end of the ninth opening, raise your hands to forehead level. Repeat the movements of closing and opening as above except now you are pulsing the upper dan tien. Keep your shoulders and elbows relaxed. Open and close nine times (Fig. 5-20).

After the ninth closing movement, inhale and relax. Exhale and bring your hands down your body with your palms facing your centerline. When your hands reach your lower dan tien, allow them to rest by the sides of your legs.

Turning the Qi Ball

Turning the Qi ball is a great way to develop Qi between your hands, open and integrate the energy pathways in the body, and develop the dan tien. Many variations facilitate cultivating and integrating Qi.

Begin in the basic stance, with your arms out in front and your hands along the midline of your body. Bring your right hand up until it is at shoulder level with your palm facing down. Bring your left hand up to the level of your middle dan tien with the palm facing up. Your palms are facing one another. Relax your elbows. You are holding the Qi ball between your hands. Maintain your axial alignment (bai hui to hui yin) and keep an even weight on each foot. Rotate your hands so that the right hand comes below and the left hand rises above. Move slowly and keep the same distance between the hands throughout

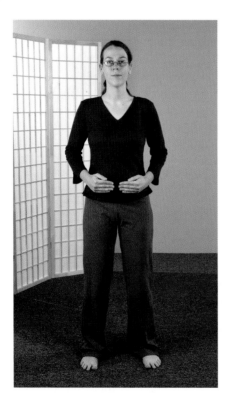

FIGURE 5-18 ■ Pulsing the lower dan tien.

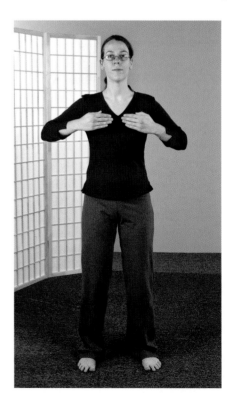

FIGURE 5-19 ■ Pulsing the middle dan tien.

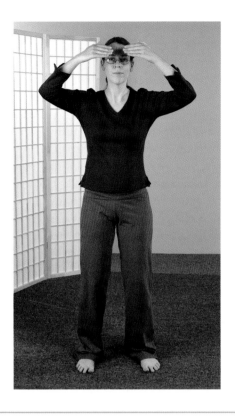

FIGURE 5-20　■　Pulsing the upper dan tien.

the rotation of the Qi ball. Feel the Qi ball as you rotate it 180 degrees. Continue to rotate the Qi ball in the other direction by rotating the hands. Continue turning the Qi ball. This is the basic Qi ball Qigong. Many variations to this exercise exist (Fig. 5-21). As you get familiar with the basic Qi ball movement, explore each variation individually. As these become familiar and you become more comfortable with each variation, combine two or more and improvise your practice. Above all, enjoy the Qi.

Body Rotation. Rotate your body as you rotate the Qi ball. As your right hand comes under the Qi ball, rotate your body to the left; as your left hand comes under the Qi ball, rotate your body to the right. The rotation is to the same side that the fingers of your lower hand point to. Do not shift your weight and keep it even on both feet.

Weight Shift. Shift your weight as you rotate the Qi ball. Your weight shifts to the same side as you rotate your body. As you are rotating your body to the left, you will shift your weight to the left. Allow

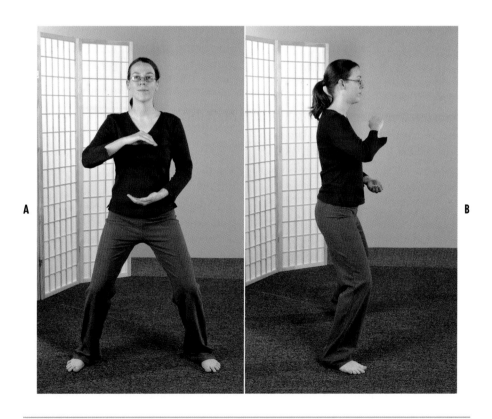

FIGURE 5-21　■　Turning the Qi ball. **A,** Front view. **B,** Side view.

the weight to shift through your pelvis. You may notice that the rotation of the Qi ball and the weight shift brings a figure-eight continuum of flow. As you shift weight, maintain the energetic alignment between bai hui and hui yin. Do not laterally flex or sway your spine. Use the Central Channel to support your axis and core.

Center to Periphery. Explore the relation of your core (dan tien) to your periphery (your hands). Play with shifting your weight to rotate the Qi ball and rotating the Qi ball to shift weight. With practice, you will continue to refine the relation of mind and Qi.

Size of Qi Ball. Change the size of the Qi ball. As you make it smaller, concentrate the energy between your hands. As the Qi ball grows, expand your energy. The main consideration is to continue to feel the Qi and keep this feeling, no matter the size of the Qi ball. Become aware of the different size of Qi ball and the change in quality of Qi. In fact, an effective way to end a Qigong practice is to concentrate the Qi between your hands then press it into the lower dan tien to store it.

Rate of Rotation. Rotating the Qi ball slowly will set the tone, energetic feel, and alignment between the external Qi (between your hands) and your internal Qi (body alignment). As this becomes established, increase your speed. Generally a weight shift will become integrated into your body as you increase your speed. If you choose a faster rate of movement, your tissues will require more blood and you can get an aerobic workout while remaining in your energetic integrity.

Height of Rotation. Rotate the Qi ball at the level of each dan tien. Include rotating the Qi ball above your head. When rotating the Qi ball over your head, tightness in your shoulders may occur. Make sure you keep your hands, elbows, and especially your shoulders relaxed. Allow the energy to descend into your lower dan tien and your feet for support.

Stand on the Earth, Support the Sky

The seemingly simple movements in "stand on the earth, support the sky" are really an exercise in feeling and moving Qi internally while drawing Qi from the earth and the heavens. Start in the basic stance with your hands by your sides. As you inhale ("inhaling heaven's Qi"), raise your arms slowly and turn your palms so they are pressing gently upward, supporting the sky. Keep your elbows and knees relaxed and slightly flexed. Hold for a moment. As you exhale, direct the Qi toward your feet and your palms. For a few moments, breathe in heaven's Qi and direct it out to your feet and palms. After a few seconds, release and let your arms come back to your sides. Center yourself for a few moments (Fig. 5-22).

Body Scan

While standing in Qigong practice or a seated meditation, imagine a white light clearing darkness or errant Qi from the body. Begin with imagining a white plane of light above the head, like an illumined pane of glass, oriented parallel to the earth. Imagine this white light healing and clearing the energy and body tissues as it slowly travels from above your head, down your body, to below your feet. An entire passage may take several minutes. Imagine vitality, light, and awareness entering as the purifying light passes through your body. Allow the sensation and mind-state of pure health and radiance fill your body, mind, and spirit. Do this as many times as you desire.

CLOSING MOVEMENTS

Your energy field should be closed after practice, and there are many ways to do this. What follows is a two-part closing.

Stand in the basic stance. Inhale, turn your palms outward, and extend your arms out to your sides until they arrive overhead and your palms face your crown. Relax your shoulders. As you exhale, bring your arms all the way back down so that your hands are in the front of your body with your palms facing your centerline. Repeat this cycle of inhaling and bringing your arms up and exhaling and bringing your arms down two more times.

Finally, massage your dan tien. Place your hands, one palm over the other palm, on your dan tien. Traditionally the right hand is over the left for men and the left hand is over the right for

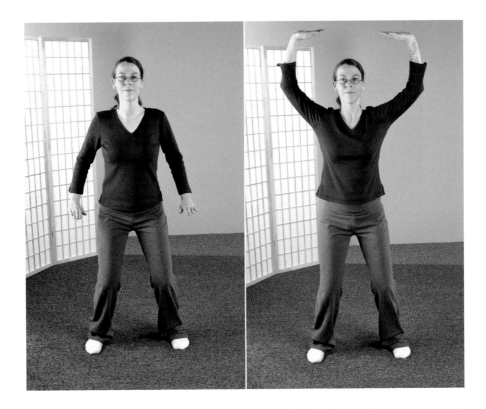

FIGURE 5-22 ▪ Merging heaven and earth.

women (Fig. 5-23). Rub your belly with your hands in a clockwise direction (up the right side, across the top of the abdomen, down the left side, and across the bottom of the abdomen). Repeat for a total of nine times. Rub nine times in a counterclockwise direction. Finish with nine circular strokes in a clockwise direction. These strokes should be firm but not hard. They should be comfortable and give you a greater sense of ease and relaxation in your core.

 BASIC SHIATSU TECHNIQUES

The shiatsu practitioner uses most of his or her own body to perform techniques during a treatment. The hands are used for palming, thumbing, and fingertip work. Also used are elbows, knees, feet, and forearms. Ki travels from the practitioner's hara out through his or her extremities to make contact and connect with the client in an effort to move, change, support, and balance the client's Ki. The goals are to alleviate tension, promote relaxation, and restore Ki imbalances.

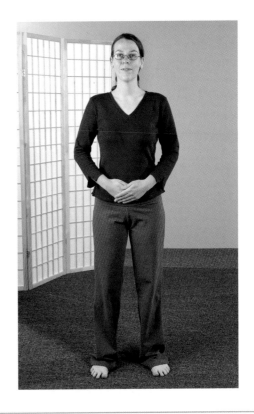

FIGURE 5-23 ▪ Massage the dan tien.

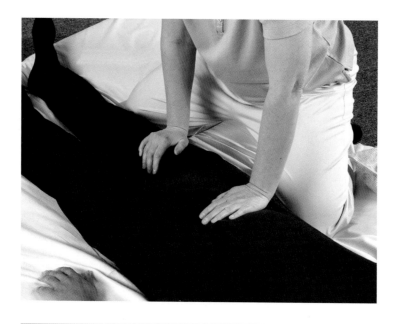

FIGURE 5-24 ▓ Leverage from the knees.

PALMING

Palming is a technique in which the practitioner uses the palm of his or her hand to apply pressure to the client's body. It is a way for the practitioner to assess the client's body. How is the client's Ki flowing? Are areas of jitsu and kyo present? What areas need more attention? What areas do not need work at all? With the Mother-hand held stationary and the Son-hand palming, the practitioner is "listening" to the client's body. Palming can also warm up the client's tissues by increasing blood flow to the area and increasing Ki flow. This can be especially helpful to warm up tissues before stretches and joint ranges of motion are performed.

Pressure is distributed evenly through the palm, and the fingers should be relaxed. The practitioner should not be grasping, simply pressing with the palm. Only enough pressure is applied to make contact and connect with the client's Ki. The pressure of palming, thumbing, and fingertip work (described below) comes from leverage, not muscle strength. The practitioner should not be using the strength of his shoulder girdle. Instead, movement should come from the practitioner's hara; leverage comes from the practitioner rising up on his knees until he achieves the amount of leverage needed. The practitioner is leaning, not pressing (Fig. 5-24).

Palming should be applied smoothly and evenly, and with the idea of sensing how the Ki should be flowing in the channels beneath the practitioner's palm. The pressure should be applied perpendicular to the client's body. Visualization of going into the bone at a 90-degree angle may be helpful; this is known as penetrating pressure. The practitioner should exhale with the client when applying pressure, then release the pressure gradually when the client inhales. Varying amounts of pressure may be used depending on the depth needed to contact the client's Ki. When the practitioner's Ki and the client's Ki connect, they can support each other and the practitioner has the opportunity to bring about necessary change in the client's Ki flow (Fig. 5-25).

5-11 THUMBING AND FINGERTIP WORK

The thumbs and fingertips are used to work more specifically on the channels and tsubo. Pressure is applied with the ball of the thumb and the pads of the fingertips. As with palming, leverage for pressure should come from the practitioner's hips, and the pressure is directed 90 degrees into the bone until Ki contact is made.

The practitioner can perform thumbing in several ways to reduce the risk of hyperextending

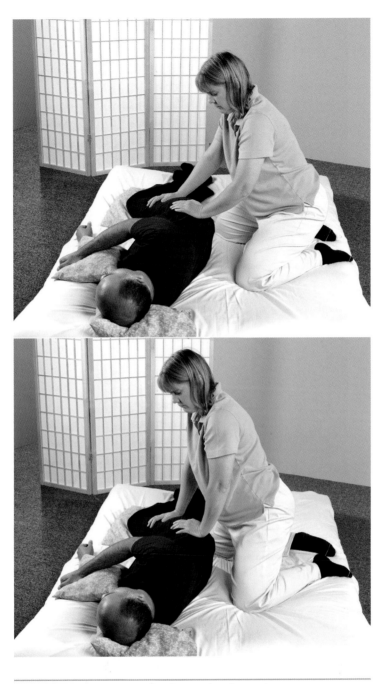

FIGURE 5-25 ■ Basic postures for using the palming technique.

the thumb. One way is called "spider thumbing." The fingers are spread out like a spider's legs to help stabilize the thumb. The thumb pad is applying the pressure; the fingers are only touching the body lightly (Fig. 5-26, *A*).

Flexed-finger thumbing involves the fingers being flexed to support the thumb. Again, the pressure is from the thumb pad; the fingers are only touching the body lightly (Fig. 5-26, *B*).

Backhand thumbing means the fingers are flexed at the metacarpophalangeal joint to provide support while the thumb pad applies pressure (Fig. 5-26, *C*).

Fingertips can be used to work areas of channels that may be too awkward to reach with the thumbs. The practitioner should not strain or hyperextend his or her fingertips or wrists while working (Fig. 5-27).

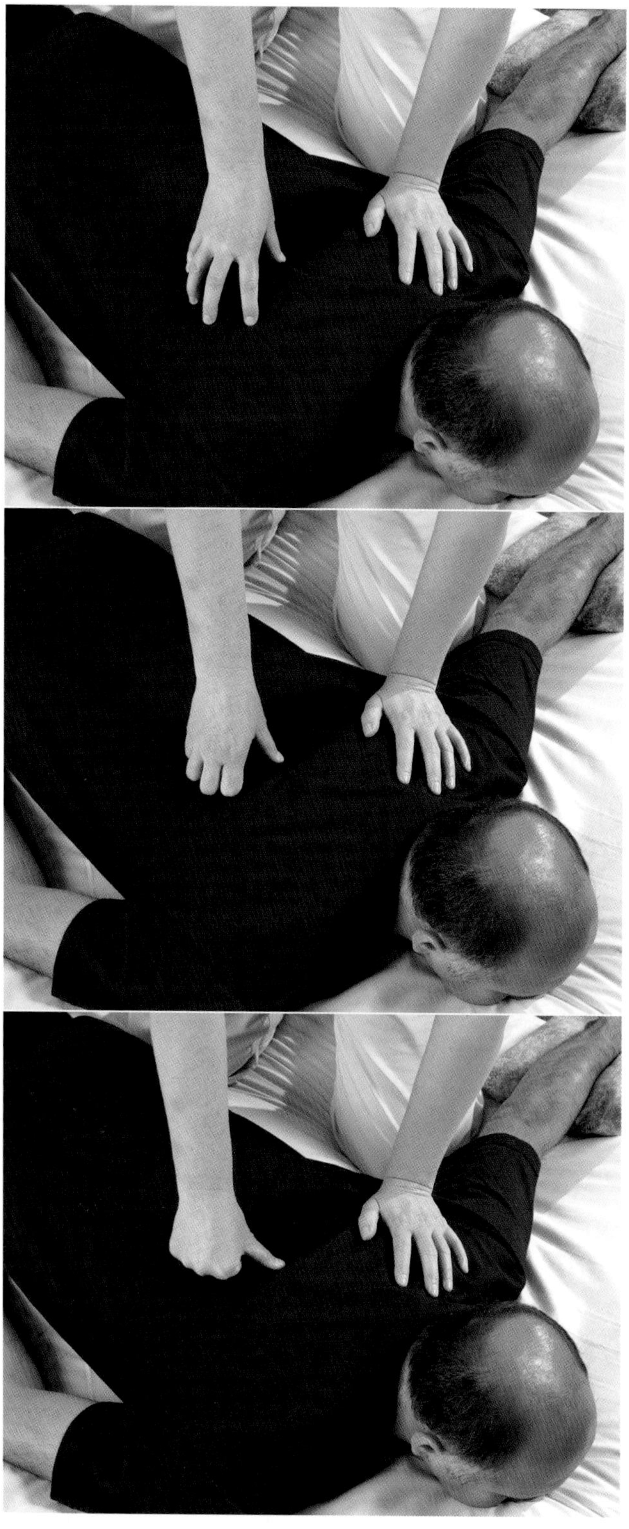

FIGURE 5-26 ■ **A,** Spider thumbing. **B,** Flexed-finger thumbing. **C,** Back-hand thumbing.

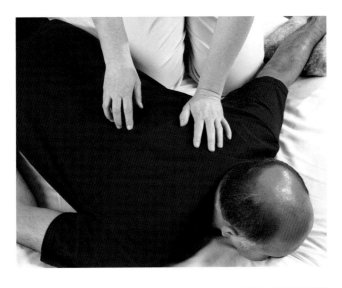

FIGURE 5-27 ■ Fingertip work.

5-12   DRAGON'S MOUTH

The "dragon's mouth," also called the "tiger's mouth," is formed between the index finger and the thumb when the thumb is abducted. The pressure is applied here. It is particularly useful for addressing the lateral sides of the client's torso, the upper trapezius, and the lateral side of the client's neck. Again, the angle of pressure applied is 90 degrees into the client's body to connect with the client's Ki. When using dragon's mouth along the client's torso, the practitioner may need to rise up on his or her knees so that leverage for pressure comes from the practitioner's hips (Fig. 5-28).

BABY DRAGON'S MOUTH

"Baby dragon's mouth" is the same as dragon's mouth except that the practitioner's index finger is flexed, so that the application of pressure comes from the thumb and knuckle. Baby dragon's mouth can be used to apply pressure down the lamina groove, working two parts of the Bladder Channel at once (Fig. 5-29).

5-13   FOREARMS

Forearms can be used by the practitioner to address a larger area than palming can cover. They can be used on the client's legs, arms, and back. Again, the intent is to provide enough pressure at

a 90-degree angle to make contact and interact with the client's Ki (Fig. 5-30).

5-14   ELBOWS

Elbows are used to provide a more penetrating pressure than from thumbing or fingertip work. Elbows can be used on the client's legs and back (Fig. 5-31).

5-15   KNEES

Like the elbows, the knees can be used to provide a deeper pressure than thumbing or fingertip work. The knees also cover a broader area than palming. Knees can be used on channels located on the client's legs, and sometimes the back and arms, if the client's arms are large enough to bear the pressure (Fig. 5-32).

5-16   FEET

The practice of barefoot shiatsu has developed many techniques performed with the feet. The feet can be used in much the same way as the palms. They can warm up areas of the client's body and provide a broad surface area for Ki connection. The feet can be applied in several ways, such as on the client's hamstrings, posterior legs, and back. When standing and using feet on the client's back, the practitioner must make sure he

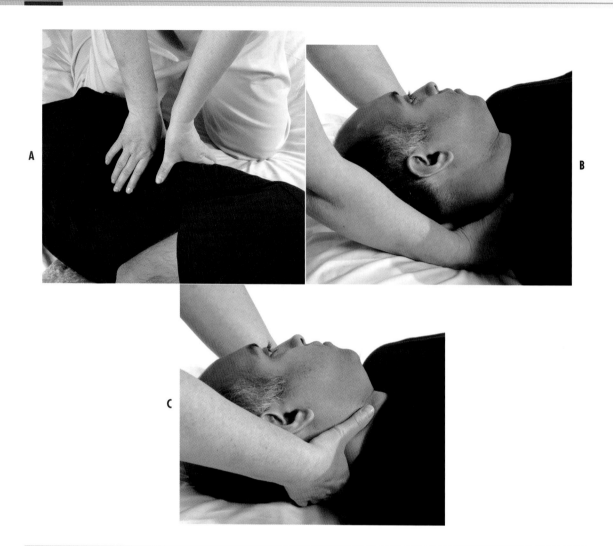

FIGURE 5-28 ■ **A,** Dragon's mouth on torso. **B,** Dragon's mouth on upper trapezius. **C,** Dragon's mouth on lateral neck.

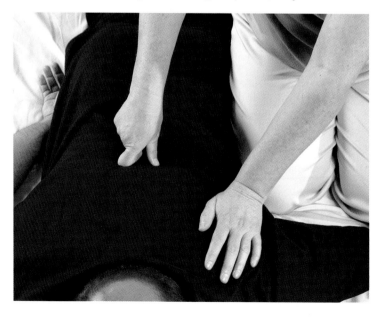

FIGURE 5-29 ■ Baby dragon's mouth.

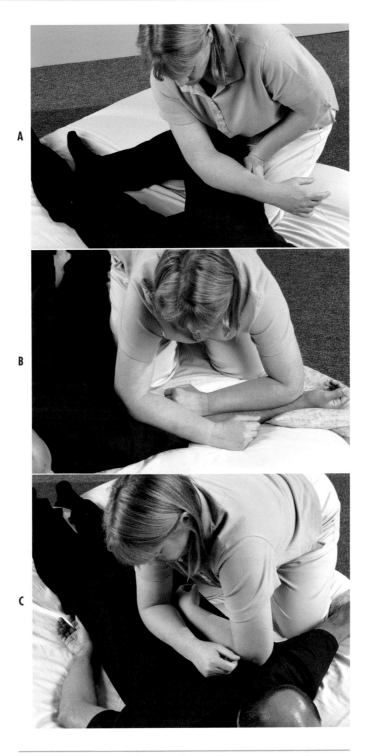

FIGURE 5-30 ■ **A,** Forearms on legs. **B,** Forearms on arms. **C,** Forearms on back.

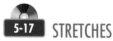

FIGURE 5-31 ■ **A,** Elbows on leg. **B,** Elbows on back.

or she is stable and grounded so as to not lose balance during these techniques (Fig. 5-33).

5-17 STRETCHES

Stretches help elongate muscles and increase the Ki flow in them. Stretches can also bring the channels closer to the surface of the body. The client's tissues should be warmed before the stretch is performed. This can be done through palming. The practitioner should perform the stretch while breathing with the client—inhaling while bring-

ing the limb into position and increasing the stretch as the client exhales. The practitioner should practice good body mechanics during stretches to prevent injury to self or his or her client. Stretches, as detailed in Chapter 6, are an excellent way to transition from one area of the client's body to another.

Many stretches can be incorporated into a shiatsu treatment, as detailed in subsequent chapters of this text. Following are some basic stretches that are useful to lengthen the arms, legs, and neck.

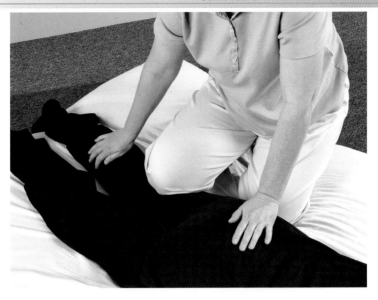

FIGURE 5-32 ■ Knees used on leg.

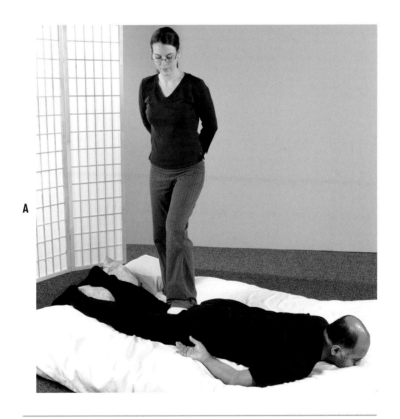

FIGURE 5-33 ■ **A,** Feet on hamstrings.   *Continued*

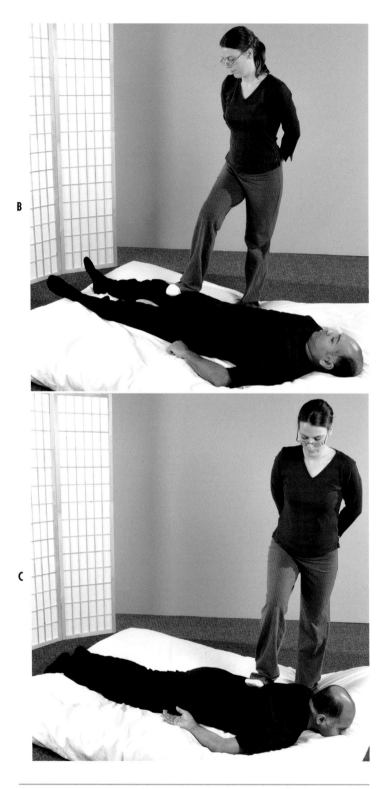

FIGURE 5-33, cont'd ■ **B,** Feet on leg. **C,** Feet on back.

Basic Arm Stretches

In the palm of the hand are two mounds of muscle. One is by the little finger and is called "little fish" in Japanese. The other is by the thumb and is called "big fish" in Japanese. They are called fish because the lighter skin of the palm and the darker skin of the back of the hand resemble how the skin of a fish changes from one part of its body to another.

In the basic arm stretches as well as other techniques, the practitioner grasps the client's big fish and little fish to move the client's arm.

Kneel perpendicularly beside the supine client. With the client's palm facing away from you, grasp the client's big fish and little fish with both hands. Gently pull the client's arm straight up for a stretch. Hold for a few seconds, then release (Fig. 5-34, *A*).

Kneel a little bit away from the supine client, at a 45-degree angle. With the client's palm facing up, grasp the client's big fish and little fish with both hands. Lean back to gently pull the client's arm into a stretch. Hold for a few seconds, then release (Fig. 5-34, *B*).

Basic Leg Stretches

Figure 4 Stretch. With the client supine, put the client's legs in a "figure 4" position—one leg laid

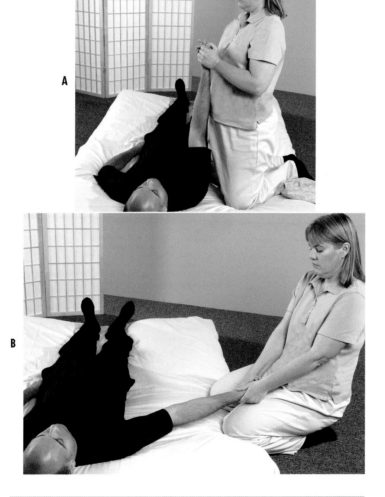

FIGURE 5-34 ■ **A,** Basic arm stretch, straight up. **B,** Basic arm stretch, 45-degree angle.

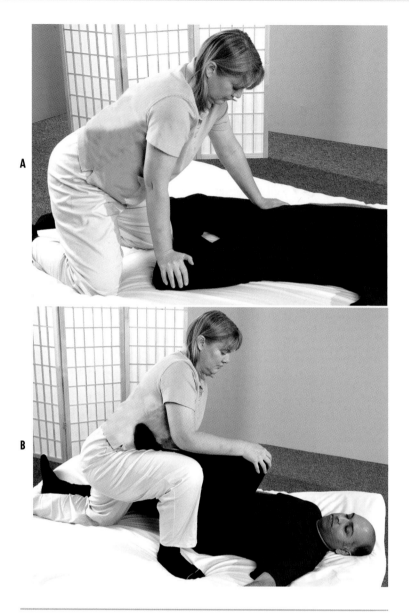

FIGURE 5-35 ▪ **A,** Figure 4 stretch. **B,** Knee-to-chest stretch.

out straight, with the knee of the other leg flexed and the sole of that foot placed against the knee of the straight leg. Kneel by the shin of the flexed leg. Place one hand on the flexed knee and the other on the opposite ASIS. Lean forward for a gentle hip stretch. Hold for a few seconds, then release. Repeat with the other leg in the figure 4 position (Fig. 5-35, *A*).

Knee-to-Chest Stretch. With the client supine, get into a lunge position facing your client's head. Tuck the client's leg into between where your leg meets your torso. Place your inside hand on your client's

hara and your outside hand on top of your client's knee. Wait for the client to inhale. When he exhales, gently lunge forward to give him a hip stretch. Hold for a few seconds, then release. Lay the client's leg out straight. Repeat on his other leg (Fig. 5-35, *B*).

Basic Neck Stretch
With the client supine, turn his head to one side. Place your inside hand on his occiput; place your outside hand on his shoulder opposite to the direction his head is turned. Gently pull on the occiput and push on the shoulder for a lateral

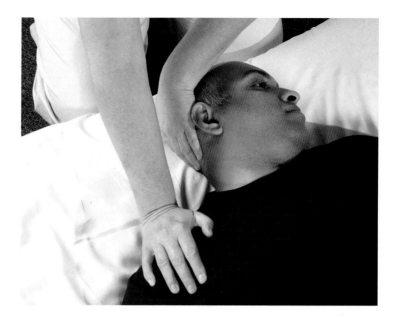

FIGURE 5-36 ■ Basic neck stretch.

neck stretch. Hold for a few seconds, then release. Center the client's head, then repeat on the other side of his neck (Fig. 5-36).

Stretch (Working) Positions

A series of stretches can also be thought of as working positions for each of the channels. When the client's body is placed in each of these positions, the channels are the most accessible for the practitioner (Fig. 5-37).

If a practitioner knows the stretch position for each channel, then the channel location does not need to be memorized. Instead, the channel becomes apparent as soon as the client is placed in the particular stretch position.

RANGE OF MOTION

Ki tends to collect and become stagnant in certain places of the body. The joints are primary sites for this occurrence. Signs of Ki stagnation are joint stiffness, pain, and limited range of motion. Performing joint range-of-motion movements can warm and loosen joints, bring blood to the area, increase nutrition within the joint by moving the synovial fluid within the joint, and increase Ki flow.

Many range-of-motion techniques can be incorporated into a shiatsu treatment, as detailed in subsequent chapters. Following are some basic range-of-motion techniques that are useful for the shoulder and hip joints. When performing joint range-of-motion techniques, the practitioner must be sure she has a wide base and is quite stable to prevent injury to himself or herself or the client.

 Shoulder Range-of-Motion Technique

With the client supine, kneel next to the client, facing his head. Place your inside hand on top of his shoulder. Grasp his wrist with your outside hand. While keeping the client's elbow flexed at 90 degrees, move his arm clockwise several times in a wide range of motion (within the client's tolerance), then move the arm counterclockwise several times in a wide range of motion (within the client's tolerance). Make sure you move your body as well; this should not be performed in a static position. Lay the arm flat. Repeat on the other arm (Fig. 5-38).

 Hip Range-of-Motion Technique

With the client supine, half-kneel by the client's legs. While supporting under her heel and under her knee, bring her leg into a flexed hip and knee position. Move your hand from under the

Text continued on p. 131

A

B

C

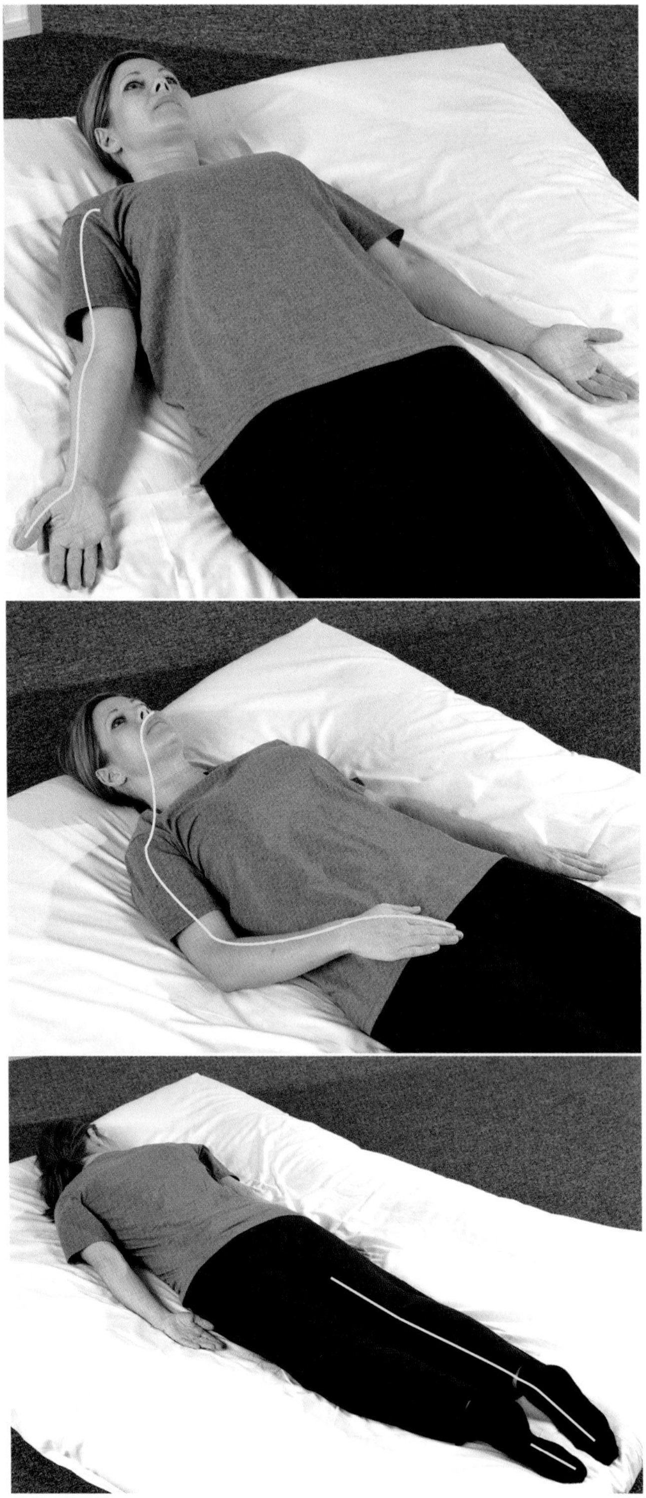

FIGURE 5-37 ■ Stretches for **A,** the Lung Channel; **B,** Large Intestine Channel; **C,** Kidney Channel.

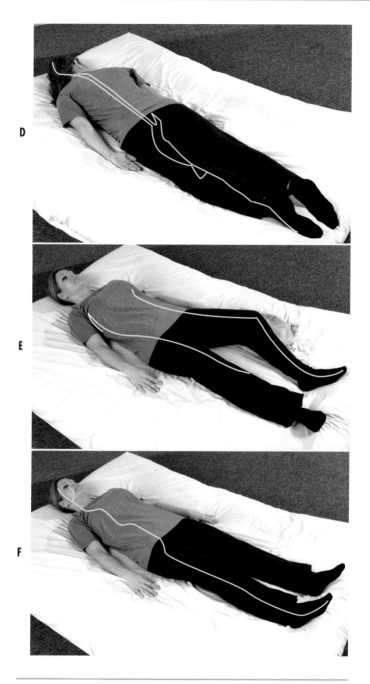

Figure 5-37, cont'd ■ Stretches for **D,** Urinary Bladder Channel; **E,** Spleen Channel; **F,** Stomach Channel. *Continued*

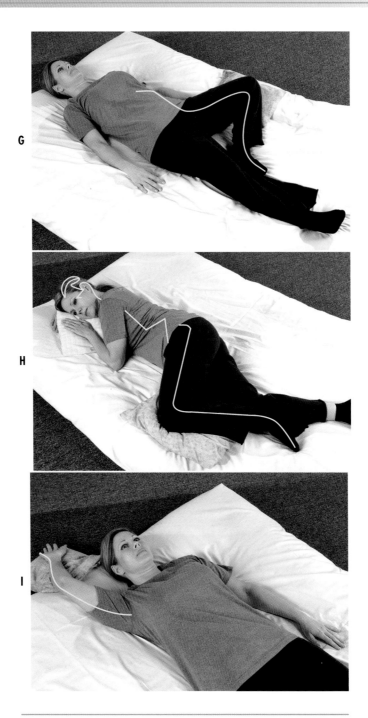

FIGURE 5-37, cont'd ■ Stretches for **G**, Liver Channel; **H**, Gallbladder Channel; **I**, Heart Channel.

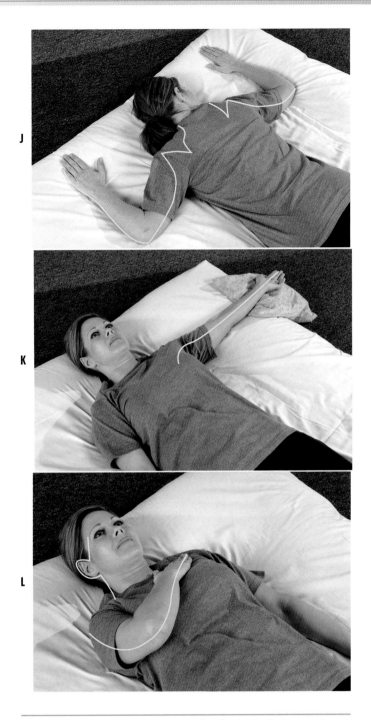

FIGURE 5-37, cont'd ■ Stretches for **J,** Small Intestine Channel; **K,** Heart Protector Channel; and **L,** Triple Heater Channel.

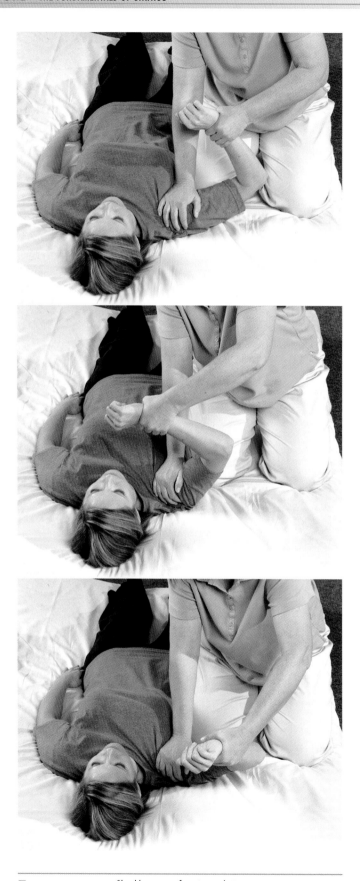

FIGURE 5-38 ■ Shoulder range-of-motion technique.

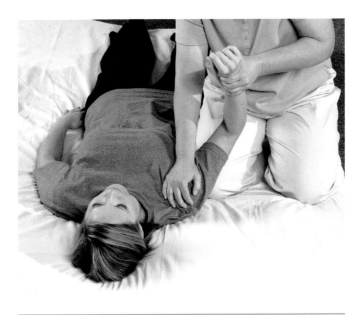

FIGURE 5-38, cont'd ■ Shoulder range-of-motion technique.

knee to on top of the knee. Use the hand on top of the knee to guide as you move her leg clockwise several times in a wide range of motion (within the client's tolerance), then move the leg counter-clockwise several times in a wide range of motion (within the client's tolerance). Make sure you move your body as well; this should not be per-formed in a static position. Repeat on the other leg (Fig. 5-39).

GENERAL PRINCIPLES OF TREATMENT

To be present, the practitioner should rely on and constantly return his awareness to correct breathing (diaphragmatic and through the nos-trils) and body alignment (incorporating balance and use of the three treasures). Connection with the client is of utmost importance. The following can serve as reminders of how to practice shiatsu and how to make the treatment as beneficial as possible:

1. Do not press; simply be there.
2. Use both hands; stay connected.
3. Be natural; be yourself.
4. Be continuous; go with the flow.
5. Be reverent of all life.

The practitioner must learn to achieve mutual trust by supporting his client physically and emotionally through thoughts, actions, and words.

 To love what you do and feel that it matters; how could anything be more fun?
~Katherine Graham

ADDRESSING JITSU AND KYO

Once the practitioner identified what is jitsu and what is kyo in the client, he must be able to balance them. At the simplest level, jitsu must be dispersed, and kyo must be supported or toned.

Because jitsu is excessive Ki or overactive Ki, another way to think of addressing Ki is that it needs to be sedated. A sensation of being pushed out by jitsu can occur because more than enough Ki is in the area, and it generally does not welcome intrusion. A more Yang approach may be neces-sary. Once the Ki is contacted, do not linger there; that would draw more Ki to the area. Instead, as soon as contact is made, release the connection,

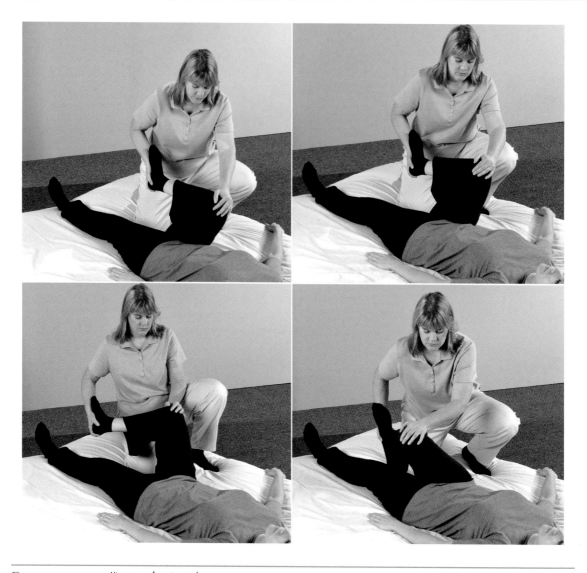

FIGURE 5-39 ■ Hip range-of-motion technique.

then penetrate again. Do this down the length of the channel until you feel the Ki flow smooth out. To assist in the dispersal or sedation, visualize the Ki moving away from the jitsu area. If a point is particularly jitsu and unyielding, apply clockwise, circular penetration with the thumb or finger into the point, then pull out with a counterclockwise, circular motion. Focus and practice are required to apply pressure for just the right length of time for sedation, and not so long that more Ki collects in the area.

If a larger area of the client's body than a channel or part of a channel is jitsu, more active techniques may be used. The massage techniques of vibration, heat-producing friction, and percussion may be useful. Through the motion of these techniques, the jitsu areas can sometimes be seen to dissolve. Range-of-motion techniques, as previously described, are extremely useful for diffusing jitsu in the joints.

Kyo tends to draw the practitioner in, and pressure may need to be applied to penetrate quite deeply before contacting Ki. The practitioner needs patience and focus because it may take time for the kyo to fill. This is more of a Yin sense—stillness and waiting. Or, the filling may occur immediately. The decisive factor is the connection between the practitioner's Ki and the client's Ki. This connection serves as a catalyst for balancing kyo. The Ki filling the kyo area is not coming from the practitioner. Rather, the practitioner draws attention to the kyo area so that the client's Ki will be drawn there.

Once the kyo has rebalanced, the practitioner should feel responsiveness and energy in the area. Continuing to penetrate once the rebalancing has occurred is not necessary. Some areas are so kyo that they are extremely painful. Simply laying a hand on the area may rebalance it. Or touch may be too painful, and tonifying the area energetically above and without touching the client may be warranted.

1. If you are not practicing any now, choose one or more self-care methods and practice them for at least 2 weeks. Keep a journal below of how you feel physically, mentally, and emotionally during this time.

2. Practice the basic shiatsu techniques every day and note your progress in becoming more skilled.

3. Practice the methods to address jitsu and kyo every day and note your progress in becoming more skilled.

4. For #2 and #3, document your practice sessions. Include the following information:
   - Recipient's name
   - Recipient's age
   - Areas you found kyo and areas you found jitsu on the recipient
   - How you addressed the areas of kyo and jitsu
   - How the recipient responded to the techniques you used

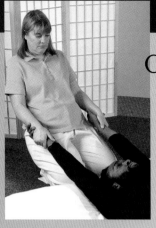

CHAPTER

6

BASIC KATA

OUTLINE

OBJECTIVES

Upon completion of this chapter, the reader will have the information necessary to do the following:
1. List the questions to ask when doing a self check-in.
2. Perform a Basic Kata.

A **kata** is a routine or protocol. Students use it in martial arts to learn moves and techniques in a logical sequence. The information in a kata is presented in such a way that every step builds on previously acquired knowledge. The **Basic Kata** in this chapter is presented in just such a way. It incorporates all the basic movements of shiatsu and shows how to work with a client in supine, prone, and side-lying positions.

The Basic Kata is presented as a focus for practice while learning techniques and as a tool to make the techniques and movements of shiatsu automatic. It is the equivalent of practicing scales when learning how to play the piano or practicing a volleyball serve over and over until it becomes second nature. Once you no longer need to concentrate consciously on body mechanics and placement of hands, thumbs, fingers, and knees, you will be able to concentrate on drawing from your acquired knowledge, and on giving yourself opportunities to develop your intuition and touch sensitivity more freely. You will have more room to develop personal style and movement in your shiatsu treatment. Your movements truly become a dance, and your treatment truly becomes therapeutic.

To make the movements of shiatsu second nature and ensure your own body mechanics, a self check-in before and during each treatment may be helpful. Body mechanics are not something that can be learned once. They require continual self-monitoring and correction. Over time, the monitoring and correction can become automatic and not necessarily require conscious effort. Until this occurs, the **self check-in** can be used as a reminder.

Basic Kata
Kata
Self Check-in

SELF CHECK-IN*

Are you comfortable? Use techniques you are comfortable with; practice uncomfortable techniques until they become comfortable. Only apply pressure to areas you can easily reach. You and your client support each other; if you are not comfortable, your client will not be comfortable either.

Are your muscles relaxed? If not, you are using unnecessary effort.

Are you grounded? Be aware of where the ground is and your own is and your client's connection with it, no matter where you are doing shiatsu. The link you have with the earth is a great source of Ki.

Are you stable? Is your supportive base as wide as you can make it? A stable base ensures that you have maximal strength, sustainability, and Ki flow. It also ensures that you have the strength and steadiness to support your client.

Are you using your hara as efficiently as possible? Your hara "illuminates" the part of the client's body you are working on ("hara headlights") and directs the way for the client's Ki. If your hara is not facing your work, you are not using your body weight. Instead, you will be "muscling into" your client.

BASIC KATA

Remember: place your hara toward your work, keep your back straight, and breathe!

 6-1 HARA TECHNIQUES

1. Sit in seiza at the right side of your client, with your head facing your client's head. Center yourself (Fig. 6-1, *A*).

*Modified from Beresford-Cooke C: Shiatsu theory and practice: a comprehensive text for the student and professional, ed. 2, Edinburgh, 2003, Churchill Livingstone.

2. Turn perpendicular to your client. Slide your left hand (Mother-hand) under your client's back. Rest your right palm (Son-hand) on his hara. Gently palpate your client's hara clockwise with your Son-hand, noting the sensations you feel in his hara (Fig. 6-1, *B*).
3. Slide your Mother-hand out from under your client's back. Gently palpate your client's hara clockwise with both hands, noting the sensations you feel in your client's hara (Fig. 6-1, *C*).

Leg Techniques in Supine Position

1. With your Mother-hand on your client's hara, palm with your Son-hand down your client's right anterior leg and foot. When you reach your client's knee, move your Mother-hand to just superior to his knee and move down so that your hara is facing your client's lower leg (Fig. 6-2, *A*).
2. Palm down the medial side of your client's left leg and foot, moving your Mother-hand and yourself down as needed to keep your hara facing your work (Fig. 6-2, *B*).
3. Perform the hip range of motion technique. Half-kneel by your client's legs. Supporting under his heel and knee, bring your client's leg into a flexed hip and knee position. Move your hand from under the knee to on top of the knee. Use the hand on top of the knee to guide as you move his leg clockwise several times in a wide range of motion (within your client's tolerance). Then move his leg counterclockwise several times in a wide range of motion (within your client's tolerance). Make sure you move your body as well; this should not be done in a static position (Fig. 6-2, *C-E*).

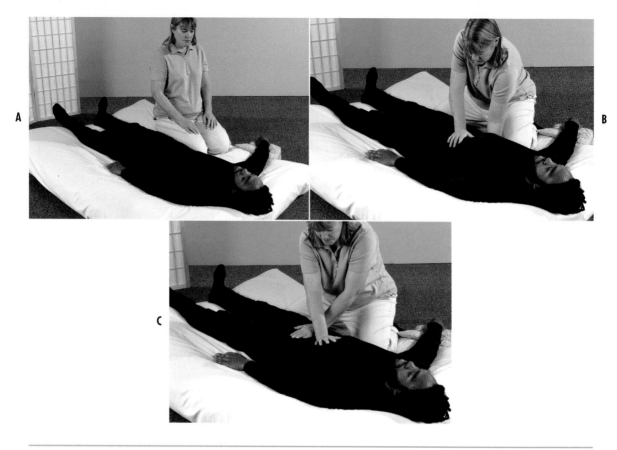

FIGURE 6-1 ▪ Hara techniques. **A,** Step 1. **B,** Step 2. **C,** Step 3.

4. Perform the knee-to-chest stretch. With your client supine, get into a lunge position facing his head. Tuck your client's leg in between your leg and torso. Place your inside hand on your client's hara and your outside hand on top of his partner's knee. Watch for your client to inhale. When he exhales, gently lunge forward to give him a hip stretch. Hold for a few seconds, then release. Lay your client's leg out straight (Fig. 6-2, *F*).

5. Bring your client's right leg into the same position as above, supporting his knee on your thigh or a small pillow (Fig. 6-2, *G*).

6. With your Mother-hand on your client's upper thigh, palm with your Son-hand down the medial side of his upper right leg. When you reach your client's knee, move your Mother-hand to his knee and palm down your client's lower leg (Fig. 6-2, *G*).

7. Lay your client's right leg out flat. Crawl to his feet.

8. While in seiza, slowly pull both your client's ankles for a hip and low back stretch. Do not lift his legs off the futon. Lifting the legs can compromise your client's back (Fig. 6-2, *H*).

9. Move to your client's left side and repeat steps 1 through 8.

10. Grasp along your client's right foot and toes. Stretch his ankle by dorsiflexing and plantarflexing it. Cup the heel in your left hand and grasp the foot along the sole with your right hand. Move the foot clockwise several times in a wide range of motion (within your client's tolerance) then move the foot counterclockwise several times in a wide range of motion (within your client's tolerance). Repeat on your client's left ankle, foot, and toes (Fig. 6-2, *I*). Lay both legs out straight.

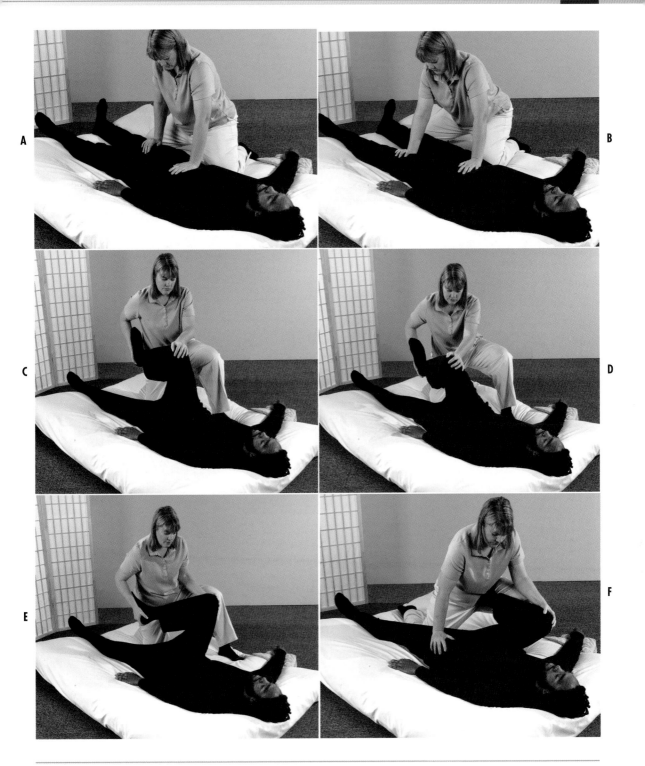

FIGURE 6-2 ■ Leg techniques in supine position. **A,** Step 1. **B,** Step 2. **C-E,** Step 3. **F,** Step 4.

Continued

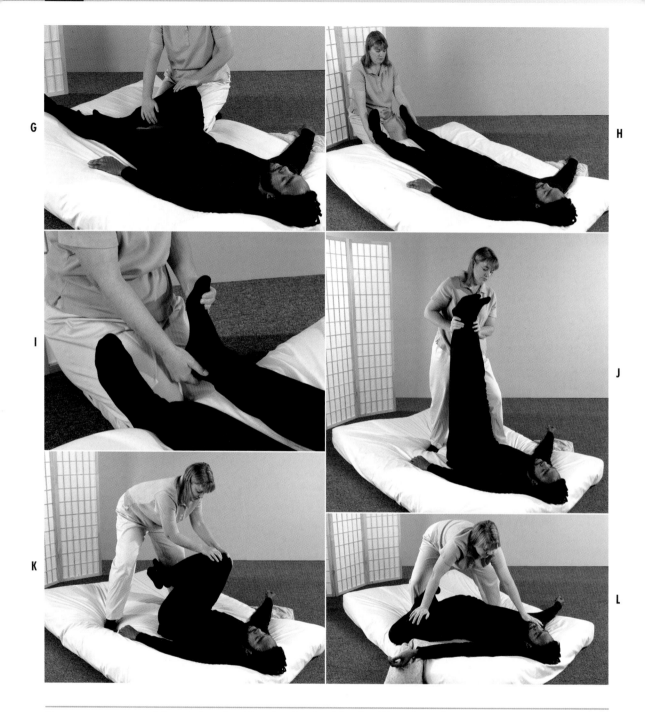

FIGURE 6-2, cont'd ■ **G,** Steps 5 and 6. **H,** Step 8. **I,** Step 10. **J,** Step 11a. **K,** Step 11b. **L,** Step 11c.

11. Perform a stretching and loosening sequence for your client's low back. ⚠ **This should only be performed on clients who do not have low back issues, such as a herniated disc.**

    a. Grasp around your client's ankles and pick up his legs. While keeping your client's legs straight, stand up. Push his straight legs forward, stepping forward as you do so. Hold for a few seconds, then release. This technique stretches your client's low back (Fig. 6-2, *J*).

    b. Flex your client's knees and place your hands on top of his knees. While keeping your client's legs together, move his legs clockwise several times in a wide range of motion (within your client's tolerance), then move the legs counterclockwise several times in a wide range of motion (within your partner's tolerance). Make sure you move your body as well; this should not be done in a static position (Fig 6-2, *K*).

    c. Push both your client's knees to one side of his body, bracing his feet inside your calf. Perform an across-the-body stretch by placing one hand on your client's shoulder and your other hand on the lateral side of your client's knee that is on top. Gently press down. Hold for a few seconds, then release. Bring your client's knees to center and repeat with his knees on the other side of his body. Lay your client's legs out straight (Fig. 6-2, *L*).

6-2 *Techniques in Side Position*

1. Place your client in a side-lying position. Place a small pillow next to his left hip. Crawl to your client's right side. Cup your right hand under his right heel and place your left hand under his right knee. Flex your client's leg, then bring your left hand out from under the knee to on top of his knee. Perform a range of motion technique. On the final turn, step across your client's bottom leg and place his flexed leg on the pillow next to his left

hip. If your client has not already done so, move his right arm over to rest in front of him. Support your client by placing small pillows between his hands to hold as well as under his head (Fig. 6-3, *A-E*).

2. Kneel close to your client's back, facing his head. Rest your right hand on your client's right shoulder and your left hand on his right scapula. Pause for a moment (Fig. 6-3, *F*).

3. Insert your arm under your client's axilla to clasp his shoulder with both of your hands, sandwiching the shoulder. Move the shoulder clockwise several times in a range of motion, then move the shoulder counterclockwise several times in a range of motion (Fig. 6-3, *G*).

4. Use both your hands to slide his right arm straight up as you move into a kneeling position perpendicular to your client. With your client's palm facing away from you, grasp Big Fish and Little Fish with both your hands. Stretch his arm gently toward the heavens (Fig. 6-3, *H*).

5. Move so that you are kneeling again at your client's back while laying his arm in front of him. While facing your client's head, perform dragon's mouth along the side of his torso. You may need to rise up on your left leg for better leverage depending on your body size and your client's body size (Fig. 6-3, *I*).

6. Move down a bit to your client's hip and perform circular kneading motions on his hip (Fig. 6-3, *J*).

7. Palm down the lateral side of your client's upper (right) leg. Palm down the medial side of his lower (left) leg. You may need to rise up on your right leg for better leverage depending on your body size and your client's body size (Fig. 6-3, *K* and *L*).

8. Bring your client out of side-lying position and back into supine position. Step across your client's bottom leg and cup his right heel with your right hand and place your left hand under his right knee. Perform a counterclockwise range of

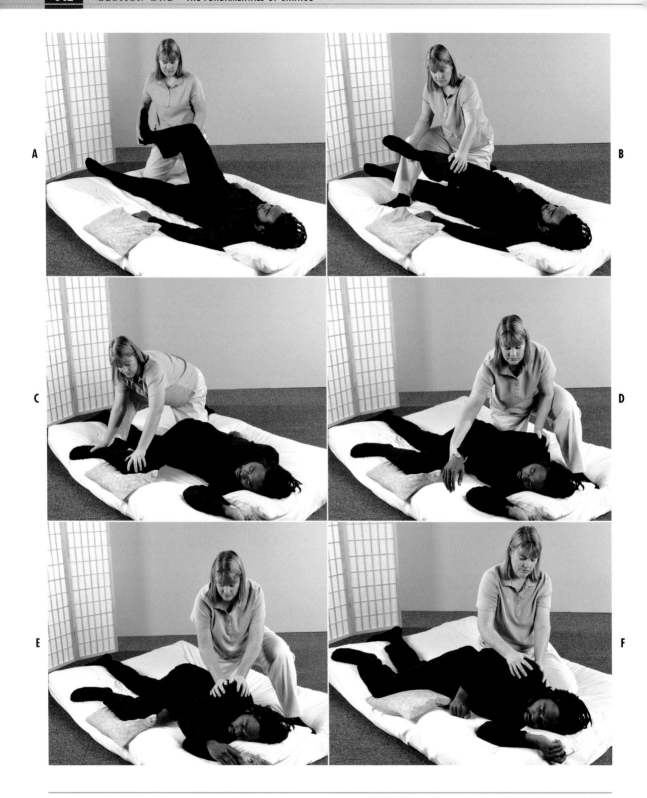

FIGURE 6-3 ■ Techniques in side-lying position. **A-E,** Step 1. **F,** Step 2.

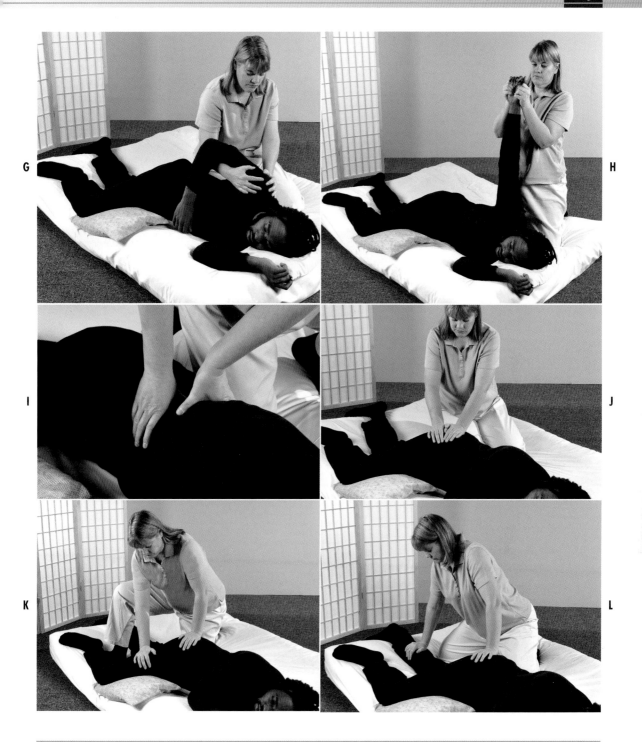

FIGURE 6-3, cont'd ■ **G,** Step 3. **H,** Step 4. **I,** Step 5. **J,** Step 6. **K** and **L,** Step 7.

Continued

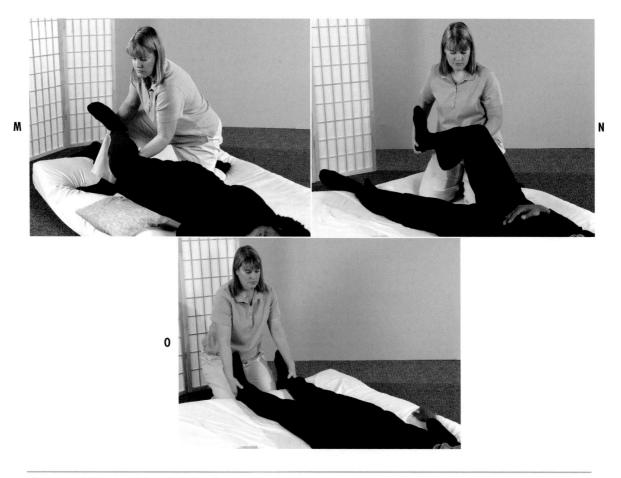

FIGURE 6-3, cont'd ■ **M-O,** Step 8.

motion technique to bring your client's leg back into supine position. Lift both his feet to straighten him out and place his right arm by the right side of the body if necessary (Fig. 6-3, *M-O*).

9. While keeping a hand on your client, crawl to his left side and repeat steps 1 through 8.

 Torso Transition

1. Stand up and straddle your client at his feet. Work your way up to your client's torso by rocking both his legs and hips and walking up at the same time (Fig. 6-4, *A-C*).

2. Kneel next to the right side of your client, facing his head. Fold your hands together and press them up gently through your client's hara and sternum (Fig. 6-4, *D*).

3. Rise up and palm and knead your client's upper pectoral muscles, starting medially and working out laterally to his shoulders (Fig. 6-4, *E*).

 Arm Techniques in Supine Position

1. Sit in seiza by your client's right arm.

2. With your right hand as Mother-hand on your client's right shoulder, grasp his wrist with your left hand. While keeping your client's elbow flexed at 90 degrees,

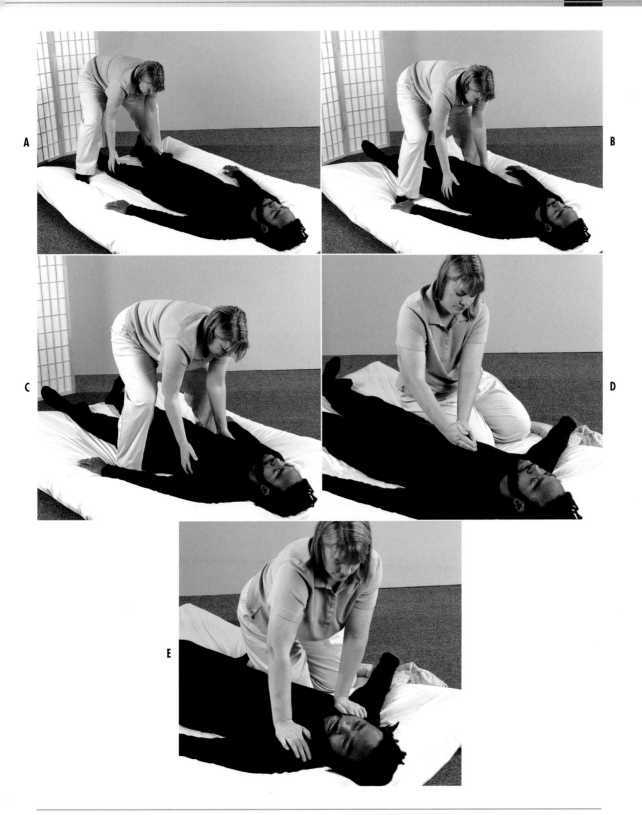

FIGURE 6-4 ■ Torso transition. **A-C,** Step 1. **D,** Step 2. **E,** Step 3.

move his arm clockwise several times in a wide range of motion (within your client's tolerance), then move his arm counterclockwise several times in a wide range of motion (within your client's tolerance). Make sure you move your body as well; this should not be done in a static position. Lay your client's arm out flat (Fig. 6-5, *A*).

3. Lay your client's right arm straight out at a 90-degree angle from his body. With your right hand as Mother-hand on your client's shoulder, palm with your left hand down the medial side of his arm and hand (Fig. 6-5, *B*).

4. Interlace your right fingers with your client's fingers and move his wrist clockwise several times in a range of motion (within your client's tolerance), then move his wrist counterclockwise several times in a range of motion (within your client's tolerance). Pull your fingers from your client's fingers slowly (Fig. 6-5, *C*).

5. Lay your client's arm palm side down along his body.

6. With your left Mother-hand on your client's shoulder, palm with your right hand down the lateral side of his arm (Fig. 6-5, *D*).

7. Turn your client's hand palm side up. Cradle his hand with your hands and knead his palm with your thumbs. Pull your fingers out slowly (Fig. 6-5, *E*).

8. Stabilize your client's wrist with your left hand. Stretch, perform range of motion, and "milk" each of his fingers with your right hand (Fig. 6-5, *F*).

9. Grasp your client's right hand with your right hand and crawl with it up to kneel at his head. Grasp your client's left hand with your left hand and bring it up toward his head. Lean back to stretch both his arms at once (Fig. 6-5, *G*).

10. Move forward, or rise up on your right leg, and toss your client's right arm onto the futon (Fig. 6-5, *H* and *I*).

11. Repeat steps 1 through 9 on your client's left arm. Move forward, or rise up on either your right or left leg, and toss both

your client's arms onto the futon (Fig. 6-5, *J* and *K*).

Neck Techniques

1. Sit in seiza at your client's head. Palm and knead his upper pectoral muscles and shoulders (Fig. 6-6, *A*).

2. Gently hold your client's head for a moment. Rest your thumbs flat across his forehead, then hold your palms and fingers over his temples (Fig. 6-6, *B*).

3. Glide up your client's posterior neck with your fingers, moving his hair out of the way if necessary (Fig. 6-6, *C*).

4. Cradle your client's occipital ridge with your fingertips (Fig. 6-6, *D*).

5. Overlap your fingers and, with your hands against your client's occipital ridge, lean back slowly with your entire body to open and stretch the cervical spine. **Only perform this technique on clients who do not have any neck issues.** Release the stretch slowly and straighten your client's head and neck into a relaxed position (Fig. 6-6, *E*).

6. Gently massage your client's face and scalp (Fig. 6-6, *F*).

7. Place your palms over your client's eyes and hold for a moment (Fig. 6-6, *G*).

8. Have your client turn over.

Back Techniques

1. Sit in seiza on your client's right side, facing his head. Center yourself.

2. Move so that you are perpendicular to your client. Palm randomly all over your client's back and gluteals (Fig. 6-7, *A*).

3. With your Mother-hand on your client's right scapula, palm with your Son-hand down the right side of your client's back and gluteals. Be careful to not put direct pressure over the spinal column. Palm with your Son-hand down the left side of your client's back and gluteals (Fig. 6-7, *B*).

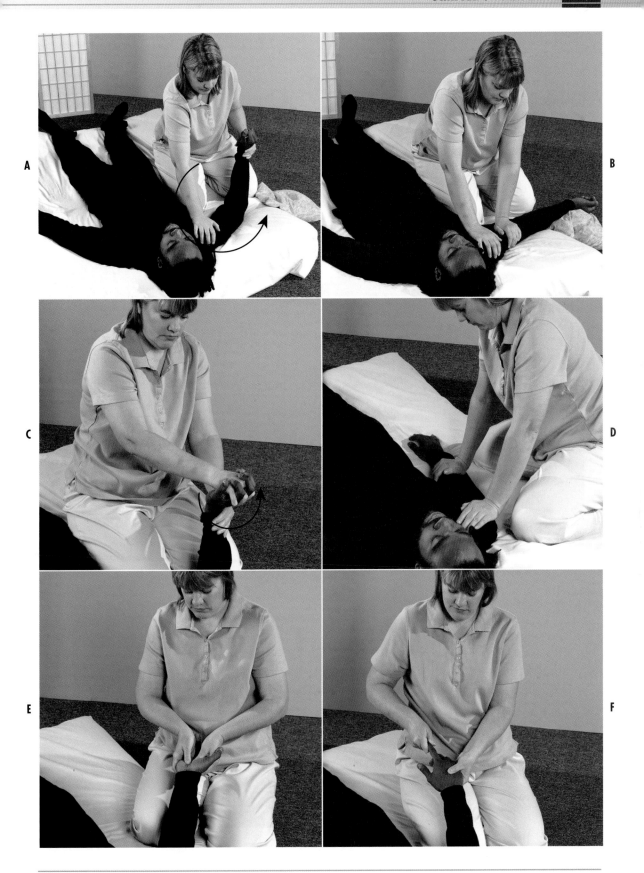

FIGURE 6-5 ■ Techniques for the arm in supine position. **A,** Step 2. **B,** Step 3. **C,** Step 4. **D,** Step 6. **E,** Step 7. **F,** Step 8.

Continued

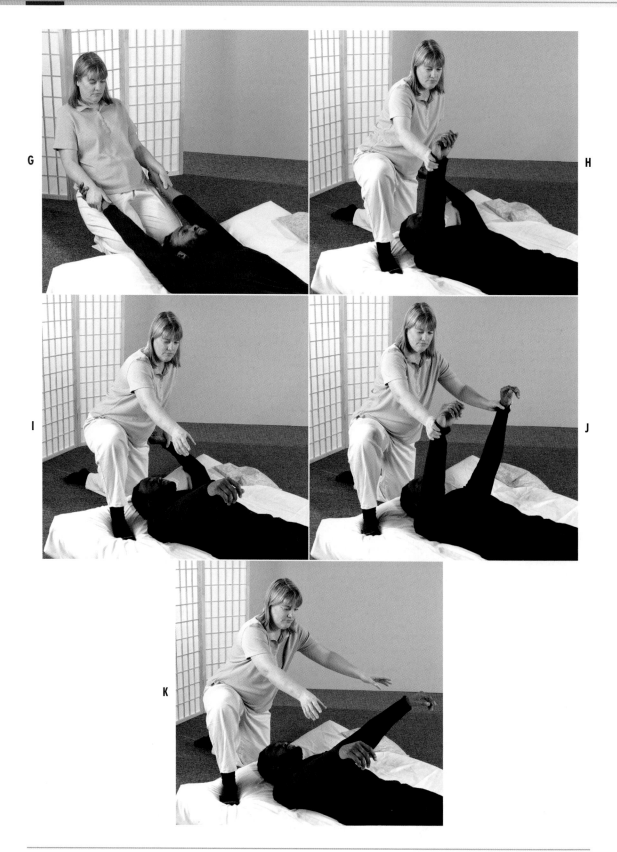

FIGURE 6-5, cont'd ■ **G,** Step 9. **H** and **I,** Step 10. **J** and **K,** Step 11.

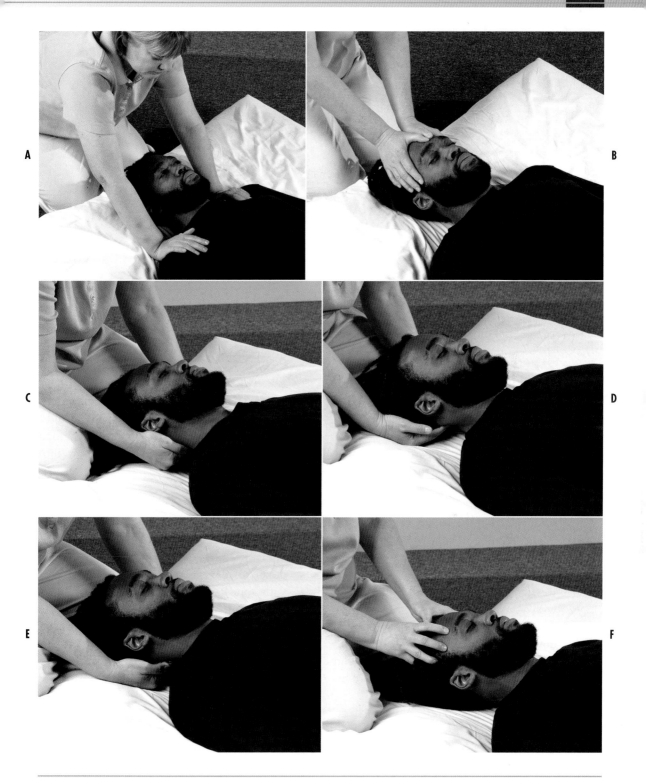

FIGURE 6-6 ■ Neck techniques. **A,** Step 1. **B,** Step 2. **C,** Step 3. **D,** Step 4. **E,** Step 5. **F,** Step 6.

Continued

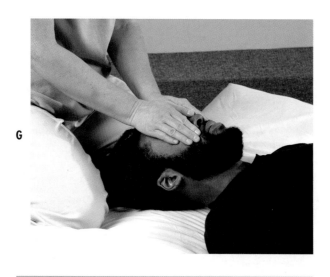

G

FIGURE 6-6, cont'd ■ **G,** Step 7.

4. With one hand on your client's left posterior iliac crest and the other hand on his right inferior angle of the scapula, slowly lean forward to perform a lumbar cross stretch. Switch so that you are making contact with the right posterior iliac crest and the left inferior angle of the scapula; repeat the stretch (Fig. 6-7, *C*).

5. While keeping a hand on your client, crawl to his head. Lean in to both shoulders and knead them (Fig. 6-7, *D*).

6. Rise up onto one knee and, while leaning with your weight forward to exert perpendicular pressure, bilaterally thumb down the lamina groove of your client's vertebrae. Come back up to his head and bilaterally thumb down the middle of his erector spinae (Fig. 6-7, *E*).

7. While keeping a hand on your client, crawl to his left side. Repeat steps 3 and 4.

8. Stand up and straddle your client with your feet outside his hips. Palm down (or use the backs of your hands) your client's erector spinae bilaterally, exerting perpendicular pressure into him (Fig. 6-7, *F*).

9. While still straddling your client, go down on one knee. Interlace your fingers and lean into each side of the sacrum, squeezing with the heels of both hands. Bring your body forward to strengthen the action and/or tuck one elbow into your leg (Fig. 6-7, *G*).

 Leg Techniques in Prone Position

1. While keeping a hand on your client, crawl down to his right gluteals and knead them with your hands or your fists (Fig. 6-8, *A*).

2. With your Mother-hand on your client's sacrum, palm down your client's right leg and foot. When you reach your client's knee, move your Mother-hand to just superior to his knee and move down so that your hara is facing his lower leg (Fig. 6-8, *B*).

3. While supporting your client's right anterior ankle with your right hand and stabilizing his sacrum with your left hand, perform a three-way quadriceps stretch. Make sure you move your body as well; these movements should not be done in a static position.

    a. Flex your client's knee and point the foot toward the center of his gluteals. Lean gently but firmly, then slide your hand toward his toes to stretch the ankle in

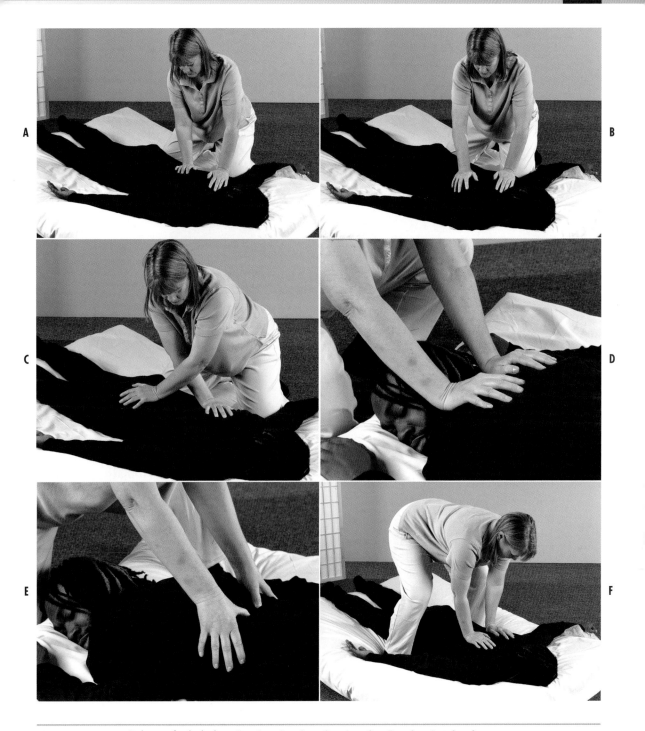

FIGURE 6-7 ■ Techniques for the back. **A,** Step 2. **B,** Step 3. **C,** Step 4. **D,** Step 5. **E,** Step 6. **F,** Step 8.   *Continued*

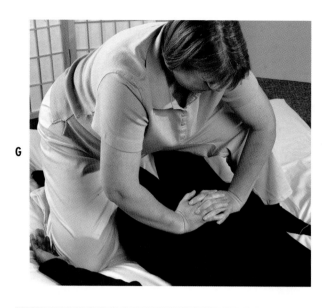

FIGURE 6-7, cont'd ▪ **G,** Step 9.

plantar flexion. Hold for a few seconds, then release (Fig. 6-8, *C*).

b. Flex your client's knee and point the foot across to his opposite gluteals. Lean gently but firmly. Hold for a few seconds, then release (Fig. 6-8, *D*).

c. Move your client's leg in a clockwise movement to perform range of motion of the leg toward you, then place it along the lateral side of his gluteals. Lean gently but firmly. Hold for a few seconds, then release (Fig. 6-8, *E*). Lay your client's leg out straight.

4. While keeping a hand on your client, crawl to his left side and repeat the three-way stretch on his left leg. Lay his leg out straight.

5. Repeat steps 1 and 2 on the left leg.

6. While keeping a hand on your client, crawl to his feet and grasp both ankles. Lean back slowly for a bilateral leg stretch (Fig. 6-8, *F*).

7. Bilaterally knead the soles of your client's feet. Place your knees into the soles of his feet (Fig. 6-8, *G* and *H*).

 FINISHING THE TREATMENT

1. Have your client turn over.

2. While keeping a hand on your client, crawl back to his hara and sit in seiza with your head facing his head.

 We are what we repeatedly do. Excellence, then, is not an act but a habit.
~Aristotle

3. Gently palpate your client's hara clockwise with both your hands, checking for changes in his hara compared with the beginning of the treatment (Fig. 6-9, *A*).

4. Gently rest your hands on your client's hara for a few moments. Let your hands rest on his hara as he inhales and exhales. After a moment, lift your hands when your client exhales (Fig. 6-9, *B*).

5. Re-center yourself (Fig. 6-9, *C*).

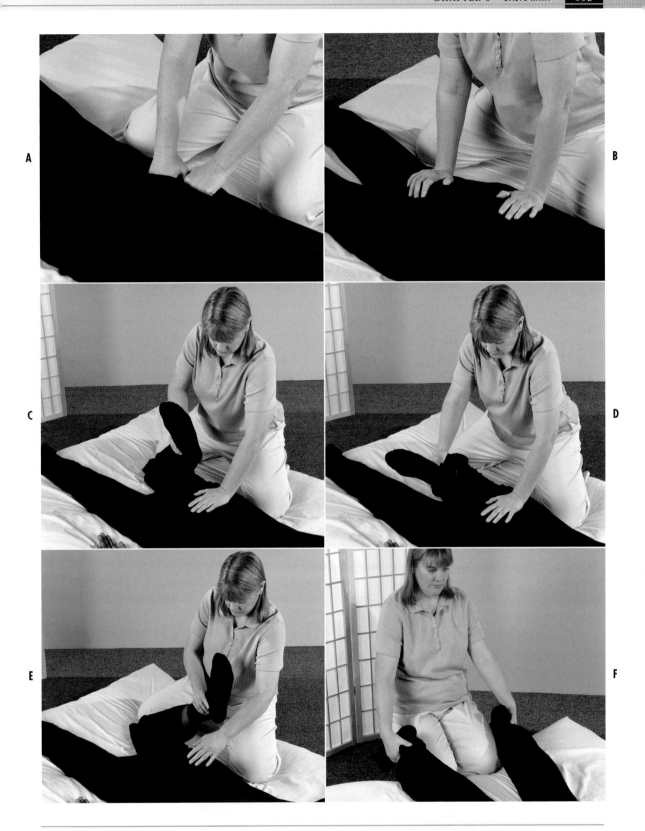

FIGURE 6-8 ■ Leg techniques in prone position. **A,** Step 1. **B,** Step 2. **C,** Step 3a. **D,** Step 3b. **E,** Step 3c. **F,** Step 6.   *Continued*

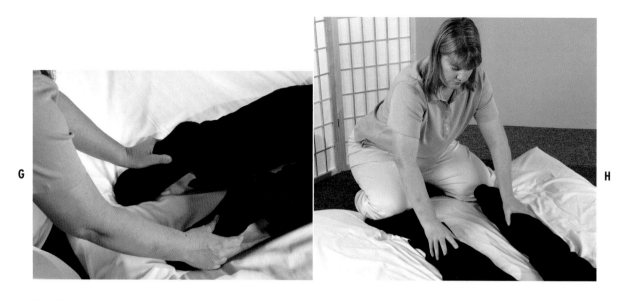

FIGURE 6-8, cont'd ■ **G** and **H,** Step 7.

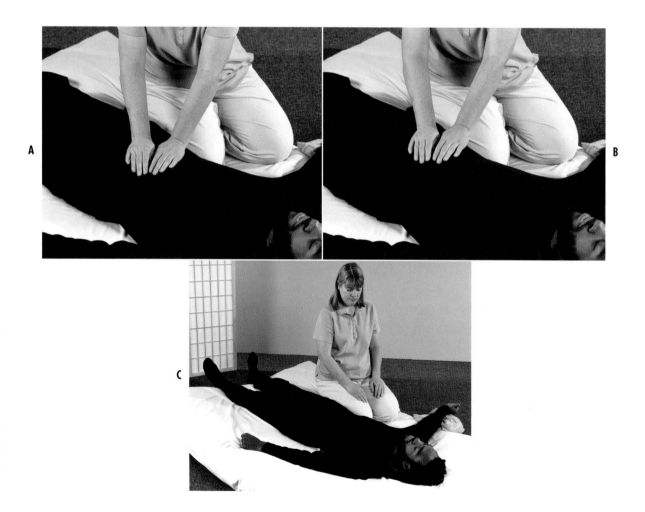

FIGURE 6-9 ■ Finishing the treatment. **A,** Step 3. **B,** Step 4. **C,** Step 5.

WORKBOOK

1. Practice the Basic Kata until you can perform it without reading it. It should become second nature. Practice on at least two clients a week. Document your practice sessions. Include the following information:

    • Recipient's name
    • Recipient's age
    • The techniques you practiced
    • How the recipient responded to the techniques you used

Practice Session 1

_____

_____

_____

_____

_____

_____

_____

_____

_____

Practice Session 2

_____

_____

_____

_____

_____

_____

_____

_____

_____

Practice Session 3

_____

_____

_____

_____

_____

_____

_____

_____

_____

_____

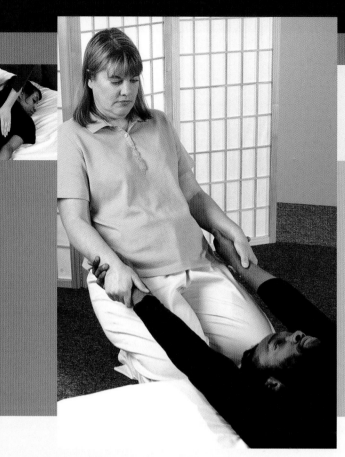

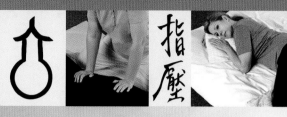

SECTION TWO

INTEGRATION OF THEORY AND PRACTICE

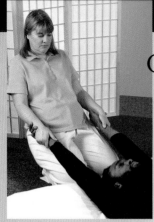

ASSESSMENTS AND THE TREATMENT SESSION

OBJECTIVES

Upon completion of this chapter, the reader will have the information necessary to do the following:

1. Explain several ways theory and practice are integrated for the shiatsu practitioner.
2. Explain each of the Four Methods of Assessment, including their use in the practice of shiatsu.
3. Perform postural and Ki assessments on clients.
4. Continue to develop touch sensitivity.
5. Perform hara assessments.
6. Determine kyo and jitsu in a client, both in the hara and elsewhere in the client's body.
7. Conduct a pretreatment interview.
8. Outline the components of the treatment session.

INTEGRATION OF THEORY AND PRACTICE

Students of shiatsu often find bridging theory and practice difficult. A misconception exists that traditional Chinese medicine is separate from the actual application of techniques. The understanding that traditional Chinese medicine is the underlying foundation of shiatsu and a wealthy resource to draw from makes the choice of which shiatsu techniques to use when treating a client much easier.

The bridge between theory and practice can be partially crossed by understanding that throughout the ages certain imbalances in the body have been discovered to present as characteristic patterns. The majority of discomforts people experience present themselves in a surprisingly small number of common imbalance patterns. Accordingly, foundational treatment methods that correspond to these patterns are available to the shiatsu practitioner. In other words, through knowledge and experience, Asian bodywork practitioners determined over time that for each of the most common imbalance patterns a

Asking	Ki Patterns	Observing	Postural Patterns
Hara Assessment	Listening	Palpating	The Four Methods

specific set of techniques can be performed, and a certain set of tsubo can be worked to alleviate discomfort (see Chapter 8). The shiatsu practitioner can use these treatments as a basis for tailoring the shiatsu session to the client's needs, then add his or her own creativity in the form of a wide variety of techniques.

The bridge between theory and practice is further crossed by the use of assessments. In traditional Chinese medicine assessments are sometimes referred to as "diagnoses." However, in Western culture, diagnosing falls under the purview of physicians and is beyond the scope of practice of shiatsu practitioners. The term *assessment* is actually closer in meaning to the traditional Chinese medicine use of the term *diagnosis.*

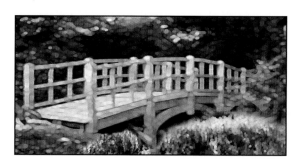

The pretreatment interview (discussed later in this chapter) gives the shiatsu practitioner a certain amount of information about the state of the client's Ki, but assessments complete the picture. The shiatsu practitioner can use assessments to determine longstanding conditions as well as what the client is experiencing in the moment. The assessments included in this chapter are all grouped under the **Four Methods** of Assessment: **listening**, **observing**, **palpating**, and **asking**.

Finally, the bridge between theory and practice is completely crossed when the shiatsu practitioner gains experience. By working conscientiously and diligently, the integration of

knowledge, intuition, and methods occurs naturally. The more the practitioner practices, the stronger and more complete the integration.

They may forget what you said, but they will never forget how you made them feel.
~Carl W. Buechner

THE FOUR METHODS

The Four Methods of Assessment used in traditional Chinese medicine are listening, observing, palpating, and asking. Although using one of these methods to determine the design of the client's treatment may be effective, the shiatsu practitioner benefits by using two, three, or all four methods. One assessment may indicate a particular imbalance that other assessments could corroborate or contradict. When using all four methods, at least three of them generally will point toward the element imbalance or discomfort pattern that the shiatsu practitioner should address during treatment.

LISTENING

During the listening assessment, the practitioner listens to what the client is saying, how she is saying it, and perhaps what the client is not saying. Although listening to what the client is saying is important, the practitioner can also open his awareness to the tone and timbre of the client's voice.

The quality of the client's voice can indicate an imbalance, either temporary or chronic, in the Five Elements. Does the client's voice seem to have a singing value (Earth)? Does she have a loud, commanding voice (Wood)? Does the client's voice sound weepy or whiny (Metal)? All

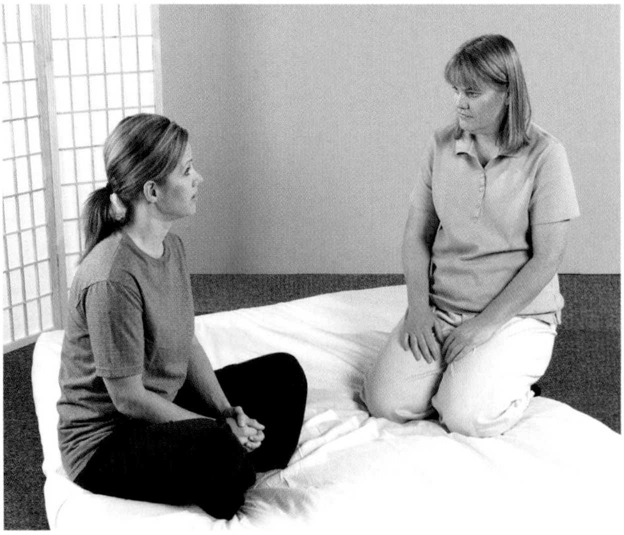

FIGURE 7-1 ■ Shiatsu practitioner interviewing a client.

these voice qualities are listed as correspondences to the Five Elements (see Chapter 3).

If her voice has a quality that is not appropriate to the words the client is saying, that discrepancy can also be a clue. For example, laughing while describing a sad event can indicate a Heart or Small Intestine Channel imbalance. The sound for Fire is laughter, and an imbalance in Heart or Small Intestine can present as inappropriate laughter. A clipped tone when describing a happy event can indicate a Liver Channel imbalance. Clipped tones are usually associated with anger, the emotion that corresponds to the Wood element. If the client's voice has a fearful undertone, a Kidney Channel imbalance may be present. Fear, of course, is associated with the Water element.

Lastly, also listen for what the client is not saying. When recounting events that can be relevant to her current state, does the client seem to leave something out? This can be a clue to her emotional state. Some things may be too painful or sad for the client to talk about, or perhaps she has a lot of anger. Be sensitive to the client's state, and if there is something the client seems to be unwilling to say, do not press her for more information. She may or may not be receptive to talking about emotions if asked. In addition, do not make assumptions about the client's emotional state if she has not disclosed this informa-

tion. Make a mental note to see if something shows up in other assessments of the client. Share information if it seems appropriate to the treatment session but always be mindful of the impact the information could have on the client. Maintain professional boundaries and stay within the scope of shiatsu practice (Fig. 7-1).

OBSERVING

The observing assessment is just what it sounds like: assessing the client for visual clues. The shiatsu practitioner can use three main categories of observation: hue of the client's face; the client's posture, body movements, and demeanor; and the client's body energy patterns.

When looking for the client's facial hue, remember that the color of the client's skin is not important. This is not a focused look at the client, but more of an unfocused extension of visual awareness of the client. Does a particular color seem to float around or radiate from the client's face? Is a color reflection present? Is there an overlay, like a transparency, of a particular color on the client's face? This skill may take some practice to acquire. Stay relaxed and be receptive, with a mind clear of thoughts.

Particular hues may indicate an imbalance in the following elements:

Red: Fire
Blue or black: Water
Green: Wood
White: Metal
Yellow: Earth

The client's posture, body movements, and demeanor all illustrate the client's Ki. Because Ki is the force behind both substance and movement, it presents in the body physically and energetically. A person who has excess Ki generally has bold movements and a loud voice, whereas someone who is deficient in Ki can be slower moving and have a weak voice. Someone whose Ki is relatively in balance stands up straight yet is relaxed. Are the client's eyes clear and face open? Is her handshake firm? Hands warm? Voice not too loud or soft? All of these are clues as to the strength and vitality of the client's Ki.

Postural and Ki Patterns

Postural patterns can be the result of Ki manifestations. Areas of the body that are sunken in are usually kyo, and areas that push outward are usually jitsu. For example, an excessive lordotic curve can indicate kyo in the lumbar erectors, or jitsu in the abdominal muscles. Shortened pectoralis major muscles draw the shoulders inward, and the chest area will be kyo. The corresponding elongated upper back muscles could then be jitsu. Scoliosis would have kyo in the chronically shortened areas and jitsu in the chronically elongated areas of the erector spinae. Interestingly, the reverse could be true: jitsu in chronically shortened areas and kyo in the chronically elongated areas. How postural patterns present is different in each individual (Fig. 7-2).

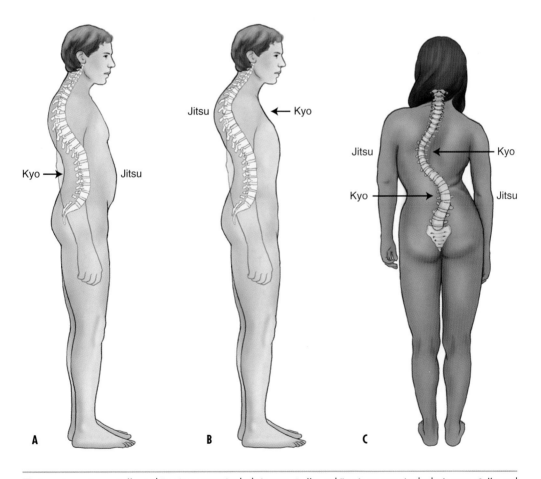

FIGURE 7-2 ■ **A,** Kyo and jitsu in an excessive lordotic curve. **B,** Kyo and jitsu in an excessive kyphotic curve. **C,** Kyo and jitsu in scoliosis.

Many times Ki energy patterns are more subtle than can initially be seen by a novice. Practice is required to see the physical and energy patterns at the same time. The energetic flow of Ki is usually superimposed on the physical presentation of a person. To see it, the shiatsu practitioner must open his awareness and use an unfocused gaze. Patience is required at first until the practitioner is able to "see" and "not see" as the same time—in other words, to see two realms of a person at once.

Is the client's Ki up or down? Is a marked difference present between the upper half of the body and the lower half? This can be observed while the client is lying on the futon or walking. Does the client plant her feet firmly? If so, she has a good Ki connection with the earth and is grounded. If the client plants her feet too firmly, then her Ki may be stagnant in the lower part of the body. If the client's feet seem to barely touch

the ground, then her Ki may not be grounded enough.

If the Ki is more in the upper half of her body, then the treatment session should begin with work on the lower half of the client's body to draw Ki downward and balance her upper and lower body. If the Ki is more in the lower half of her body, then the treatment session should begin with work on the upper half of the client's body to draw Ki upward and balance her upper and lower body. The client's Ki may not appear to be excessively up or down; it may already be balanced between her upper and lower body (Fig. 7-3).

Is the client's Ki stronger on the left or the right side of her body? If it appears weaker on one side, begin the treatment session on that side. By drawing Ki to that side, the two sides balance out (Fig. 7-4).

Is the client's Ki strong or weak? This assessment gives the practitioner an idea of what tech-

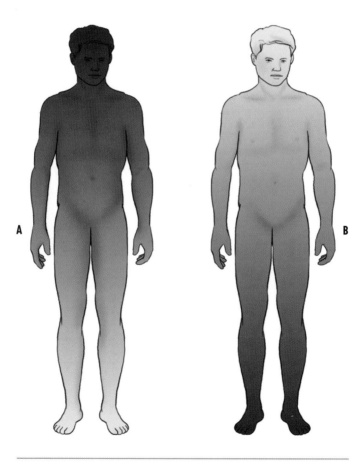

FIGURE 7-3 ■ **A,** Ki "up" in the body. **B,** Ki "down" in the body.

niques to use and how vigorously they should be applied. For example, someone with a robust Ki may respond well to strong stretches and wide range-of-motion techniques. The practitioner's Ki may easily connect with the client's Ki, thus giving the practitioner more time during the treatment session to use a variety of techniques.

Someone with weak Ki may require fewer vigorous techniques. In fact, dynamic techniques may fatigue the client. Instead, the practitioner may need to spend more time using static touch to connect with the client's Ki and use his own Ki to support her Ki. The treatment could be at a slow pace, one of meeting the client where he is in the moment and offering human-to-human contact for support.

Does the client's Ki seem to spiral through her body? This is quite common. People tend to have a dominant foot; they lead their walking pattern with it. The accompanying arm swinging tends to cause a spiral action of movement through the body and often causes a spiral Ki pattern. Clients with this pattern often respond favorably to across-the-body stretches (see Chapters 6 and 8). These stretches unwind tight muscles, tendons, and ligaments and unwind habitual Ki patterns. Client Ki can spiral for reasons other than dominant foot gait, such as scoliosis, injury, muscle tightness, and structural misalignment. Determining whether the client has any contraindications to across-the-body stretches is important, such as a herniated disc, before performing them (Fig. 7-5).

Is the Ki flowing or is it blocked? This can be seen while the client is lying on the futon or walking. Does her body seem to move freely? If

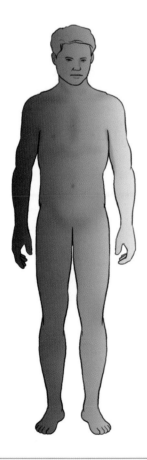

FIGURE 7-4 ■ Ki stronger on one side of the body than the other.

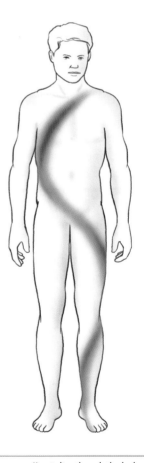

FIGURE 7-5 ■ Ki spiraling through the body.

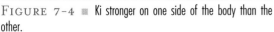

not, where does movement seem to be stuck? This is an indication of where the Ki is blocked and therefore stagnant.

If areas of the client's body have blocked Ki, then techniques to disperse the Ki should be used. Anywhere blockage is present has a corresponding area of Ki deficiency. These areas should be toned or supported.

If the Ki patterns are not immediately apparent, the practitioner should close his eyes, take a deep breath, relax, and look again. Observing with relaxed attention, seeing and not seeing at the same time, and seeing two realms of a person at once are all ways of saying the shiatsu practitioner is using intuition to connect his Ki with the client's Ki.

The shiatsu practitioner should not scrutinize the client or overanalyze what he sees. Overthinking blocks the intuition. Instead, the initial reaction usually is correct because it is intuitive. Practice is necessary to trust intuition. If, however, after a few attempts the practitioner is still unsure, he should guess. Guessing is the gateway to intuition.

PALPATING

Palpation means to assess by touch. By making contact through mindful touch, or palpation, with the intent of connecting practitioner Ki with client Ki, areas of focus can be determined for the treatment session. Although the other assessments—listening, seeing and asking—help complete the picture of the client, the palpating assessment gives the most complete view of the client and the client's needs for the immediate treatment session. In fact, even if no other assessment is performed, the palpating assessment is suited to giving the practitioner all the information needed to formulate and carry out a client-centered treatment.

By being relaxed and centered and opening his awareness, the shiatsu practitioner can get a good sense of Ki flow and blockages in the client's body. Kyo and jitsu can be assessed merely by physical contact with the client in larger regions of her body such as the shoulders, hips, stomach, and back. Specific channels also can be assessed. An entire channel may be kyo or jitsu, or just part of the channel can be kyo and another part jitsu. More formalized methods of assessing kyo and

jitsu can also be used. One is the **hara assessment** described later.

Through practice, the shiatsu practitioner develops touch sensitivity and a reliance on intuition. The practitioner palpates while relaxed, centered, and having an open, accepting mind. Palms and fingertips can initially be used. As expertise is gained, the forearms, knees, and soles of the feet can also be used to palpate. The intent is for the practitioner's Ki to connect with the client's Ki, so a light to moderate pressure, perpendicular to her body should be used. The practitioner waits for the client's Ki to rise up to meet his Ki. Intuition can then be used to determine if the area is kyo or jitsu. Range-of-motion assessments also can be performed to determine if the Ki in the joints is stagnant or freely flowing.

Palpation assessments are used in two main ways. One is as an initial assessment to design a treatment focused on the client's Ki patterns. The other is an ongoing assessment. As the practitioner performs shiatsu, he is continually assessing kyo and jitsu to learn when an area has changed. Once a kyo area has "filled," the practitioner moves on. The longer contact is made in an area, the more the client's Ki is drawn to the area, resulting in the danger of "overfilling" an area and having it turn jitsu. Jitsu areas need to be dispersed and usually worked quickly so that the Ki will keep moving and not re-collect in the area. Kyo areas generally are worked first and longer to draw Ki away from jitsu areas.

Areas that are neither kyo nor jitsu (balanced) do not need to be addressed specifically; they can simply be palmed. If these areas are worked, more of the client's Ki is drawn to the area, resulting in a chance that the area will become jitsu. Instead, note balanced areas, then move on.

 7-1 *Hara Assessment*

The hara is the center of the practitioner's gravity and the center of all movement. It is also the origin of palpatory communication for both the practitioner and the client. The hara is where the channels are closest to the surface of the body and where they are most easily palpated. Hara assessment is one of many assessments that impart information to the practitioner regarding the state of the client's Ki, which is a reflection of her physical, emotional, and mental states. This information can thus provide a focus for treatment.

Assessment of the hara can be done in many different ways; each Asian bodywork modality has its own particular method. One simple method to assess the channels in the hara has its origins in Zen shiatsu and is taught by Pauline Sasaki, a prominent teacher of Zen shiatsu. With this method, the practitioner determines the client's most jitsu and most kyo channels in the moment. The practitioner then tailors the treatment to the client's needs by balancing these two channels. Jitsu is dispersed and kyo is supported. All channels, of course, can be addressed during a shiatsu treatment. However, by focusing on the most jitsu and the most kyo channels, any minor imbalances of Ki in the other channels also become balanced.

Location of the Hara

The superior borders of the hara are at the inferior portion of the rib cage. The inferior borders are located at the anterior iliac crests, down to the pubic crest. The hara is centered at the navel.

Assessment and Routine

The routine of shiatsu practice must become completely automatic. Thinking too hard about it can interfere with the assessment, which should be done quickly. By contacting the Ki in the hara, the shiatsu practitioner is already changing the Ki in the client's channels. Repetitive hara assessments on the client may only end up confusing the practitioner; every time the hara is assessed, the channels change.

Before assessing the hara, perform a body scan to assess your own physical, emotional, and mental states. Ensure these states are kept separate from what is assessed in the client.

To be as open and receptive as possible during the hara assessment, stay relaxed and keep your mind clear throughout the process. If you maintained your boundaries, stayed relaxed, and were attentive during the hara assessment, you should not question your findings. Assess as many haras as you can to develop intuition as a shiatsu practitioner.

 7-2 *Hara Assessment Areas and Positioning**

The following is a summary of the assessment areas of the hara and proper positioning of the hands and fingers (Figs. 7-6 and 7-7):

Heart: Over the solar plexus, in a depression just below the xiphoid process. Palpate with one or two fingers vertically at a 45-degree angle (Fig. 7-8).

Gallbladder: In the right upper quadrant of the hara, just under the ribs in a small pocket between Heart and Liver. Palpate with two fingers horizontally at a 45-degree angle (Fig. 7-9).

Liver: In the right upper quadrant of the hara, just under the ribs in a wide area between Gallbladder and Lung. Palpate with three or four fingers horizontally at a 60-degree angle (Fig. 7-10).

Lung: Lung has two assessment areas: the most lateral areas in the upper hara just above the waist and just anterior to the eleventh pair of ribs. Palpate with three fingers vertically at an 80- to 90-degree angle (Fig. 7-11).

Stomach: In the left upper quadrant of the hara, just under the ribs (and over the actual stomach organ) between Heart and Triple Heater. Palpate with three fingers vertically at a 45-degree angle (Fig. 7-12).

Triple Heater: In the left upper quadrant of the hara, just under the ribs in a small pocket between Stomach and Lung. Palpate with two fingers horizontally at a 50- to 60-degree angle (Fig. 7-13).

Heart Protector: In the upper hara, on the midline between Heart and the navel. Palpate with two fingers vertically at an 80- to 90-degree angle (Fig. 7-14).

Spleen: In a circle around the navel. Palpate with all five fingers, forming a circle around the navel, or a flat palm over the navel (Fig. 7-15).

*Modified from Beresford-Cooke C: *Shiatsu theory and practice: a comprehensive text for the student and professional*, ed. 2, Edinburgh, 2003, Churchill Livingstone.

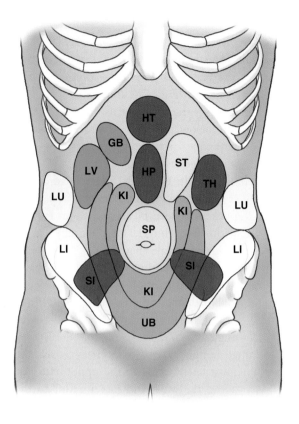

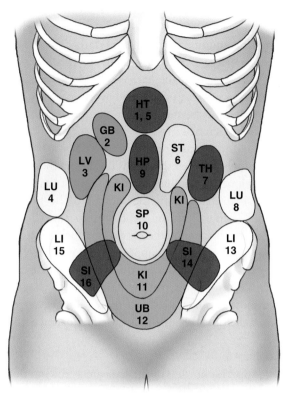

FIGURE 7-6 ▦ Hara assessment areas.

FIGURE 7-7 ▦ Proper sequence of the hara assessment routine.

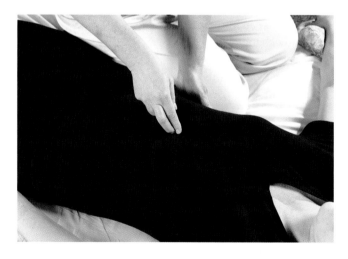

FIGURE 7-8 ▦ Proper hand position for Heart hara assessment.

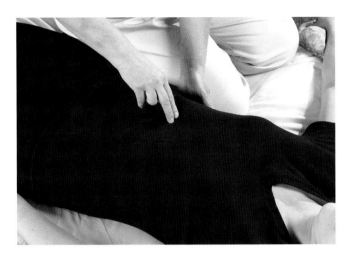

FIGURE 7-9 ■ Proper hand position for Gallbladder hara assessment.

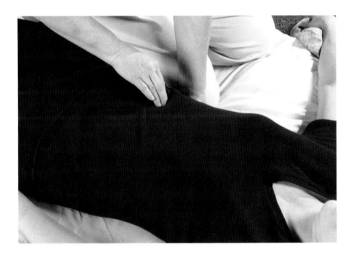

FIGURE 7-10 ■ Proper hand position for Liver hara assessment.

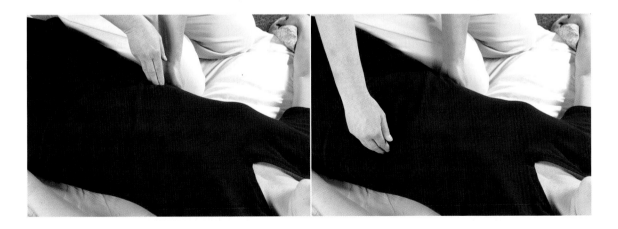

FIGURE 7-11 ■ Proper hand position for Lung hara assessment.

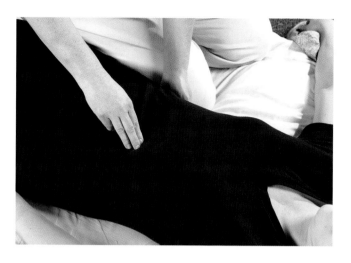

FIGURE 7-12 ■ Proper hand position for Stomach hara assessment.

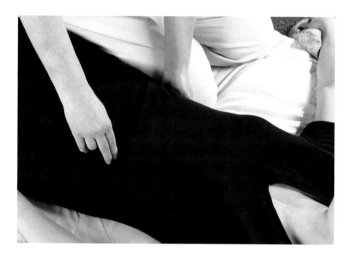

FIGURE 7-13 ■ Proper hand position for Triple Heater hara assessment.

Kidney: In the lower hara, at the curve of the belly. It is $1/2$ to 1 inch inferior to Spleen and $1/2$ inch superior to Urinary Bladder. It forms a U around Spleen assessment area and along the border of the rectus abdominis. Palpate with three to four fingers horizontally along the midline at a 45-degree angle (Fig. 7-16).

Urinary Bladder: At the edge of the lower hara, $1/2$ inch superior to the pubis and $1/2$ inch inferior to Kidney; it forms a U around the Kidney assessment area. Palpate with three or four fingers horizontally at a 90-degree angle (Fig. 7-17).

Large Intestine: Large Intestine has two assessment areas; both are in the lower hara inside the medial angle of the ilium. Palpate with three or four fingers or the medial side of the hand vertically at a 45-degree angle (Fig. 7-18).

Small Intestine: Small Intestine has two assessment areas: they are in the lower hara, successively intersecting Lung, Urinary Bladder, and Kidney. Together they create an upside down V from the navel. Palpate with four fingers or the medial side of the hand vertically at an 80-degree angle (Fig. 7-19).

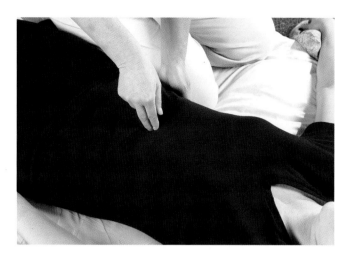

FIGURE 7-14 ■ Proper hand position for Heart Protector hara assessment.

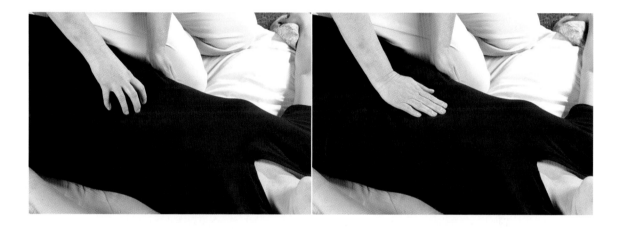

FIGURE 7-15 ■ Proper hand position for Spleen hara assessment.

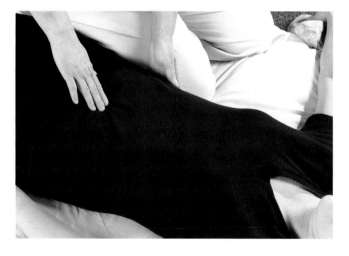

FIGURE 7-16 ■ Proper hand position for Kidney hara assessment.

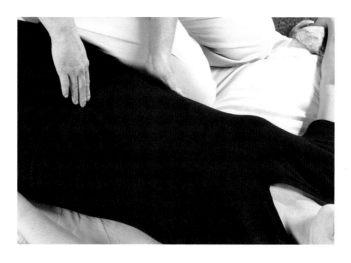

FIGURE 7-17   ■   Proper hand position for Urinary Bladder hara assessment.

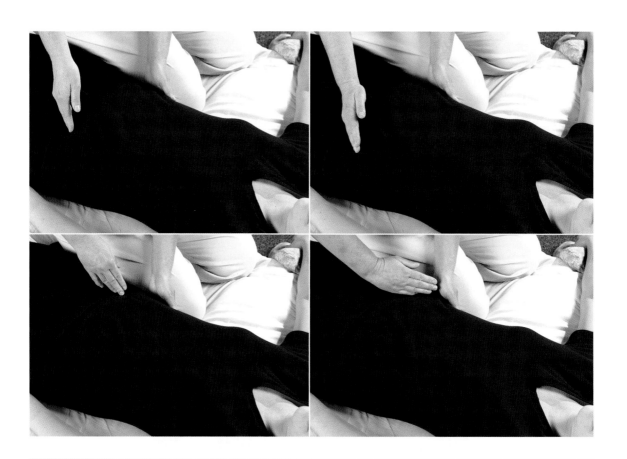

FIGURE 7-18   ■   Proper hand position for Large Intestine hara assessment.

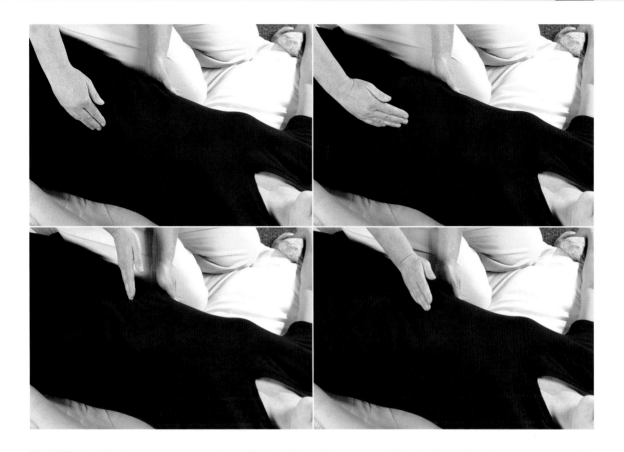

FIGURE 7-19 ■ Proper hand position for Small Intestine hara assessment.

Routine*

The following routine should be used when assessing a client's hara:

- Sit in seiza beside your client, facing her head.
- Relax; breathe into your own hara; and observe your own physical, emotional, and mental states. Note how your Ki feels in your body.
- Clear your mind and bring your focus to your client. Make yourself as receptive as possible.
- Use both hands to outline your client's hara.
- Keep one hand on an assessment area as the Mother-hand.
- Use one, two, three, or four fingertips together, depending on the size of your

fingers and the size of the assessment area. You can use the medial side of your hand for some assessment areas. Use light pressure; your client's Ki is close to the surface.

- Follow the proper sequence.
- Remember: do not overthink; trust your intuition.

Determining Most Jitsu and Kyo Channels*

When performing a hara assessment, the practitioner does not deliberately look for the most jitsu and the most kyo channels. Instead, the most jitsu and kyo channels at that moment present themselves.

The most jitsu channel is usually more obvious than the most kyo channel. Resilience or some type of reaction may be felt in the assessment

*Modified from Beresford-Cooke C: *Shiatsu theory and practice: a comprehensive text for the student and professional,* ed. 2, Edinburgh, 2003, Churchill Livingstone.

*Modified from Beresford-Cooke C: *Shiatsu theory and practice: a comprehensive text for the student and professional,* ed. 2, Edinburgh, 2003, Churchill Livingstone.

area, or heat, pulsing, or tingling may be felt in the fingers. Jitsu areas often feel raised and tight and as if they are pushing your fingers away.

Kyo, on the other hand, may be more difficult to find. Its depletion of Ki tends to make it hidden and harder to detect. Kyo tends to feel hollow, as though you are being drawn into the area.

However, jitsu and kyo have an inherent connection. Because an overabundance of Ki in one channel means diminished Ki in another channel, these channels are linked. The quickest way to find the most kyo assessment area is to hold jitsu lightly with your fingertips and palpate the other assessment areas until a connection is felt. The connection feels differently for everyone. Some of the ways shiatsu practitioners have felt this connection include the following:

- An "electric" sensation passing between their two hands
- The jitsu area decreasing while the kyo area increases
- A deep sense of just "knowing"

If you are not sure you have found the most jitsu channel or most kyo channel, relax and bring awareness into your hara before you try assessing once again. If you truly are not sure, guess. As previously mentioned, guessing is the gateway to intuition. Also, the two channels within an element should not be kyo and jitsu. If the hara assessment indicates, for example, Stomach kyo and Spleen jitsu, this is a false reading and the hara assessment should be performed again. Remember the Creation and Control Cycles of the Five Elements. If an element is out of balance then that can cause a corresponding imbalance in another element. Because they are linked, the channels within an element should be somewhat reflective of each other (both balanced, both kyo, or both jitsu), not opposite of each (one kyo and one jitsu). Do not perform the hara assessment more than twice. Remember, by palpating the assessment areas in the client's hara, the Ki in her channels will be changed.

ASKING

The asking assessment can consist of two parts: an intake form (also known as a pretreatment form or health history form) and the pretreatment session interview. The asking assessment serves two purposes: (1) to get information about the

client's state and any conditions she may have that could influence the design of treatment, and (2) to establish a connection with the client. The shiatsu practitioner can learn about the client and have an interchange that can establish trust. This is important; a shiatsu treatment, as in any bodywork treatment, is only effective if the client trusts the practitioner.

The dynamic of the asking assessment therefore is significant. It begins with the shiatsu practitioner greeting the client and introducing himself. A firm handshake and good eye contact are essential. The simple question, "How are you today?" begins the asking assessment. The shiatsu practitioner should listen to the client attentively. As the client gives information about herself, the practitioner should restate anything he is unsure of to clarify the information.

The following is a list of questions to ask the client to get as complete a picture of the client as possible and to have a good framework for designing the treatment session. Many of these questions can be asked on an intake form. Follow up by asking the client for clarification as needed.

- How do you feel right now?
- Do you have any areas of discomfort, such as pain, tightness, stiffness, or limited joint movement? Please describe the location and quality of the discomfort. (The answers can be clues to kyo and jitsu areas of the body and where the client's Ki is stagnant or blocked.)
- How long have you had this discomfort? (Chronic conditions present Ki patterns differently than do acute conditions.)
- Do you know what caused the discomfort? If so, what was it?
- What have you done so far to relieve this discomfort? What have the results been?
- Have you had any major illnesses recently? (This can be a clue to the client's overall Ki strength, vulnerability of a particular element, or any physical limitations the client has.)
- Have you had any accidents recently? (Again, this can be a clue to the client's overall Ki strength, vulnerability of a particular element, or any physical limitations the client has.)

- Have you had any surgeries recently? (Again, this can be a clue to the client's overall Ki strength, vulnerability of a particular element, or any physical limitations the client has.)
- Are you taking any medications? If so, what are the effects and side effects? (This is important to know in case the client is taking a medication, such as an analgesic, that can interfere with her ability to sense pressure.)
- Are you prone to any illnesses? (These can indicate imbalances in particular elements. See Chapter 8.)
- Does your body tend to run hot or cold? (This could be an indicator of robust or deficient Ki.)
- What type of exercise do you do, and how often do you do it? (This can give an overall view of whether the client keeps her Ki moving or if it is stagnant. It can also indicate certain elements that may need to be addressed. For example, if the client exercises excessively, Wood could be jitsu; if the client does not exercise, Earth could be jitsu.)
- How much fluid do you drink each day? (If the client has a low fluid intake, the Water Element—Bladder and Kidney Channels—could be affected.)
- How is your diet? (Whether the client has a balanced diet can have direct effects. For example, a diet high in fat, dairy, and sugar can produce Dampness, which can show up in the Stomach and Spleen Channels.)
- Do you crave particular types of food? (These are indicators of element imbalances. For example, craving sugar is an Earth Element indicator, craving salty foods is a Water Element indicator, and craving sour foods is a Wood Element indicator.)
- How is your digestion? (If the client's digestive processes are not regular, that can indicate a Metal Element issue and show up in the Large Intestine Channel.)
- How are your sleep patterns? (If the client has trouble falling asleep, staying asleep, or waking up repeatedly throughout the night, that indicates a disturbed Shen. Heart and Heart Protector Channels may need to be addressed.)
- What are your energy patterns throughout the day? Is your energy up at certain times and down at other times? (These times can indicate imbalances in certain channels. See Chapter 3.)

THE TREATMENT SESSION

The treatment session is the culmination of theory and practice. It is the actuality of knowledge and technique combined. How the session is designed makes the difference between the shiatsu practitioner helping the client create change and the session not being useful to the client. Thoughtfulness on the part of the practitioner and attention to detail can make the client's experience positive as well as therapeutic.

As discussed in the asking assessment, greeting the client with good eye contact and a firm handshake is important. When talking to the client, use reflective listening; impart to the client that you are taking an active interest in her needs.

Based on the information the practitioner receives from the client, whether through the intake form or the Four Methods of Assessment, the treatment session must be planned for the client's needs, not the practitioner's. The treatment itself can be simple or complex; it can encompass only a few techniques or myriad skills; it can be short in length or it can take a few hours. No recipe exists for exactly how shiatsu treatment is performed. However, every shiatsu treatment must have the practitioner's undivided attention on the client and the intention for therapeutic change.

After the treatment, offer the client water and check to see how she is feeling. Listening to valuable feedback about how she feels and what techniques worked or did not work for her is vital. You can use this information for future treatment sessions with the client. You also can make suggestions, within the scope of practice of shiatsu, that can help her continue to make progress. More information on these suggestions is found in Chapter 8.

1. Practice the unfocused gaze of seeing and not seeing at the same time to determine facial hues and Ki patterns on several partners.

2. Practice determining Ki patterns on partners by using a sheet. Have your partner lie down on the futon. Flutter a sheet up and let it lay gently over the person. Do not adjust the sheet in any way. Based on the folds and shadows on the sheet, see the postural patterns in your partner. Try this with your partner lying both supine and prone.

3. For at least 2 weeks, keep a separate journal of postural patterns seen on various people. Imitate those postural patterns yourself to get a sense of how they feel. At the end of 2 weeks, review your journal to see your progress in assessing postural patterns.

4. In the following diagram, label each assessment area and color it with its corresponding color. Write in the numbers for the sequence of the hara assessment.

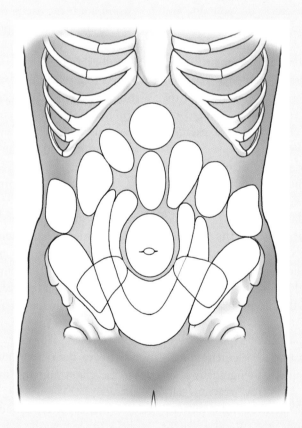

5. Practice hara assessments until the routine comes naturally. Keep a journal of your progress in determining jitsu and kyo.

    _____

    _____

    _____

    _____

    _____

    _____

    _____

    _____

6. Design an intake form in the space below based on questions to ask during the asking assessment.

7. Practice interviewing as many different partners as you can.

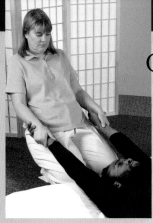

CHAPTER

8 ADDRESSING IMBALANCES IN THE FIVE ELEMENTS

Cora Jacobson
Sandra K. Anderson

OUTLINE

OBJECTIVES

Upon completion of this chapter, the reader will have the information necessary to do the following:

1. Explain the importance of moving beyond the Basic Kata.
2. Describe the symptoms of imbalances in each of the Five Elements.
3. List questions to ask a client to determine an imbalance in one or more of the Five Elements.
4. Perform a treatment, including specific work on one or more channels.
5. List recommendations for self-care for clients who have an imbalance in one or more of the Five Elements.
6. Document the treatment session.

The Basic Kata is a way for students to learn proper body mechanics and the primary techniques used to perform shiatsu. It is a routine that is practiced over and over until the techniques and body mechanics become second nature. But the Basic Kata is not meant to be a "one size fits all" treatment given to all clients. Instead, with the integration of theory and practice, the next step in the development of a shiatsu practitioner is the formulation of client-centered treatments. Client-centered treatments include not only assessing the client's needs but using the results of the assessments to decide on and carry out work on specific channels.

Information on each of the Five Elements and their associated organs and channels is presented to help the student develop a client treatment plan based on channel imbalances. This, along with information the practitioner receives from the client from the Four Methods of Assessment, is meant as a way to enrich the experience of shiatsu and assist students in developing their personal styles of performing treatments.

Channels do not necessarily need to be worked from start to finish in one continuous movement. Working each channel from beginning to end may, in fact, interrupt the fluidity of the treatment. As long as the channel is completely addressed in the session, it can be worked

Key Terms

Addressing Channels
Assessment Questions

Client Self-Care

Imbalance

Symptoms

in sections that follow the flow of the treatment the shiatsu practitioner has designed.

Each of the following channels is presented in segments that reflect the regions of the body in which it is found. These segments are designed so that the student can decide how to include work on specific channels while moving efficiently and easily around the client's body. This way, the student can create a unique way of working with each client. Students should practice incorporating specific channel work as much as possible to ensure fluidity of treatment.

Which parts of the practitioner's body to use when working channels is not specified. Only the terms Mother-hand and Son-hand are used so that the student can use his or her own originality or ingenuity in addressing channels. The student may choose to use his or her palms, thumbs, fingers, or forearms—whatever works best.

METAL ELEMENT: LUNG AND LARGE INTESTINE

The Metal element represents the body's exchange with its environment and is responsible for the ability to receive and let go. The Lungs take in air and the Large Intestine prepares waste for elimination from the body, but the Metal element has influence over many other processes. The skin is able to absorb and excrete; this body tissue is therefore associated with Metal. In terms of the emotions, the concept of "letting go" relates to the process of grieving.

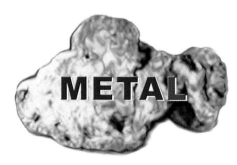

SYMPTOMS OF METAL ELEMENT IMBALANCE

When the Metal element is out of balance, symptoms may include respiratory problems, constipation, and skin disorders. A person may have frequent colds, nasal congestion, and a sore or tickly throat. Chronic skin conditions such as psoriasis or eczema tend to relate to the Lung, whereas acne or boils are eliminative and therefore are symptoms of a Large Intestine imbalance. Dryness is the climate for Metal, and dry skin, or even a lack of sweating, indicates a Metal imbalance. Sometimes the descending energy of Metal is not dispersing fluids from the upper part of the body, and the nose and eyes may be watery. Any sort of breathing difficulty, such as asthma or stuffiness, is associated with a Lung imbalance.

When someone experiences a loss of a loved one, the Metal element is affected. Grief is a natural process during such times, but when Metal is not in balance the grieving process becomes unproductive. When a person cannot stop grieving, or is unable to grieve at all, the Metal element should be addressed.

Metal is also associated with structure and the ability to be detail oriented. Imbalances may be indicated by either the overwhelming need to have everything in its place or the inability to keep things neat and orderly. As with any of the psychologic effects of an imbalance, either too much or not enough indicates disharmony.

The intake of Ki is a vital part of the Metal element. When Lung is in balance, it takes in the Air Ki to be mixed with the Food Ki that is sent up from the Spleen. If Lung is not able to receive the Air Ki, the person may feel, in addition to the symptoms discussed, a lack of vitality and a sense of disconnection from the world around him or her. The person may have difficulty taking in new experiences or appreciating what is taken in through the senses. Just as the skin provides a physical border for the body, Metal provides a psychologic border. When Metal is out of balance

177

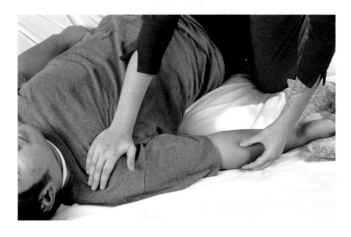

FIGURE 8-1 ■ Lung Channel being addressed in supine position.

the person may have difficulty relating to others, and feelings of isolation or depression may result.

ASSESSMENT QUESTIONS

- How is your breathing?
- How is your elimination?
- How do you feel about new experiences?
- Do you have any skin disorders or discomfort?
- Do you smoke?
- Are you organized?
- How often do you get colds?
- Do you crave spicy or pungent foods (e.g., garlic, ginger, strong cheeses)?

HOW TO ADDRESS LUNG CHANNEL

The working position for Lung Channel is with the client's arm lying palm up, at approximately a 45-degree angle from the side of his body. Lung begins at the point LU-1 in the anterior shoulder area, an ideal location for the practitioner's Mother-hand. The channel runs down along the anterior (Yin) aspect of the arm. In the upper arm Lung is on the edge of biceps brachii and in the forearm it is against the radius. The last point on the Lung channel is LU-11, on the outside edge of the thumbnail. The practitioner should be facing the arm, with one knee near the client's shoulder and the other near his hand (Fig. 8-1).

HOW TO ADDRESS LARGE INTESTINE CHANNEL

For Large Intestine working position, the practitioner places the client's hand over his Large Intes-

tine assessment area in the hara, on the belly just above the hip bone. The client's elbow is pointing out to the side, and the practitioner lines up her hara with the client's elbow. The practitioner's has a wide stance, with one knee near the client's shoulder and one knee near his hand. In this position, the practitioner works only the part of the Large Intestine channel that is on the arm. The neck and face are addressed in a different position. To begin working up the arm place your Mother-hand on the client's shoulder or hold the tsubo LI-4 in your hand. (To use LI-4 with your Mother-hand, the client's arm may need to be moved so that your thigh is supporting his hand. The angle of the elbow stays the same, at approximately 90 degrees.) The Large Intestine Channel begins with LI-1, on the edge of the index fingernail (thumb side) and runs up the arm. With your Son-hand, work up the channel on the posterior (Yang) aspect of the arm up to LI-16, in the hollow on top of the shoulder just posterior to the acromioclavicular joint (Fig. 8-2).

To work Large Intestine in the neck and face, sit in seiza at the client's head. Turn your client's head slightly to one side, supporting his head with your Mother-hand. Your Son-hand begins at LI-16 on the shoulder and works up the client's shoulder to the neck, crossing sternocleidomastoid and the mandible, to end at LI-20 at the outside corner of the nose (Fig. 8-3).

CLIENT SELF-CARE FOR METAL IMBALANCE

- Perform breathing exercises.
- Organize a closet or drawer.

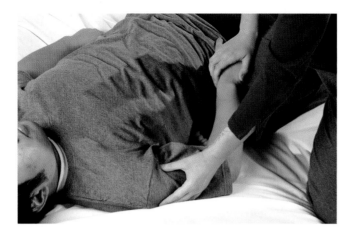

FIGURE 8-2 ■ Large Intestine Channel being addressed in the arm.

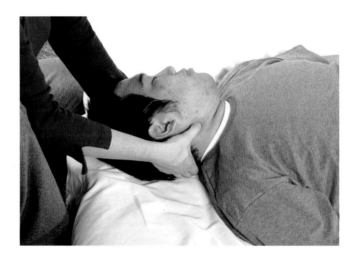

FIGURE 8-3 ■ Large Intestine Channel being addressed in the neck and face.

■ Get rid of clothes that aren't being worn.
■ Perform gentle, regular exercise.
■ Allow self to cry.
■ Avoid smoke and polluted air.

death. The body tissue of Water is the bones, the deepest part of the body. Water relates to a person's "backbone," or foundation, and to the nervous system.

WATER ELEMENT: KIDNEY AND URINARY BLADDER

8-2

The Water element houses the spark of life and is like a germinating seed in the winter. Water is the potential, or impetus, for any action a person takes or thinks about taking. The Kidney stores the essence of the body, which is used throughout a person's lifetime, until it leaves at the time of

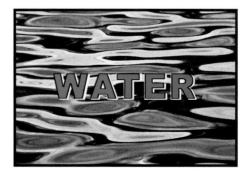

SYMPTOMS OF WATER ELEMENT IMBALANCE

When Water is out of balance a wide variety of symptoms may be present. Physically, the Kidneys and Urinary Bladder function to purify the body. Any sort of kidney or urinary disorder is indicative of a Water imbalance, such as kidney stones or urinary tract infections. Hormones of all types provide the body's cells with impetus to carry out their functions, and any hormone disorders are related to a Water imbalance. The growth process in children is governed by Water, and problems in this area are attributed to a Water disharmony. The reproductive system, especially for men, is under the control of the Water element, and sexual problems such as impotence can result from a Water disharmony. Bone issues such as arthritis and osteoporosis may be present. A Water imbalance may also cause tooth problems; teeth are part of the bones. The lower back, particularly near the kidneys, may be sore or painful. The ears are the sense organ of Water, and hearing problems and ringing in the ears are considered Water issues.

The Water connection to the backbone relates to a person's willpower and determination. When Water is out of balance, the person may be unable to initiate action. He or she may want to get something done, but does not have the drive to get up and do it. Fatigue is commonly associated with Water, as is susceptibility to stress.

The emotion for the Water element is fear. A certain amount of fear is natural and healthy because it helps keep a person safe. In a Water imbalance this may show up as anxiety, tension, or phobias. Fear may be related to the lack of drive described above; the person wants to act but is afraid to do something. Just as important as excessive fear is a lack of fear. With this type of Water imbalance, someone may be drawn to activities such as extreme sports, racing cars, and horror movies.

Water is extremely adaptable. Left alone to pool, it is deep and calm; in a storm, water becomes forceful and even aggressive. This aspect of Water provides a person with willpower and latent strength. When Water is out of balance, the person may want to "pool" his or her resources by spending quiet time alone. Conversely, a person may have difficulty being alone and strive to spend all his or her time surrounded by others to avoid the depths of the self. Balanced Water requires a certain amount of quiet time for reflection and the development of willpower. Too much quiet time is like a never-ending winter, with no chance for the new growth of spring. When the person does not have enough Water time, action may take place but the seeds did not germinate properly and the harvest may be poor.

ASSESSMENT QUESTIONS

- Do you have any back pain or discomfort?
- How is your hearing?
- How are your bones?
- Do you have a history of kidney or urinary tract problems?
- Do you have any hormone disorders?
- How do you feel about spending time alone?
- Do you crave salty foods (e.g., processed foods, potato chips, seaweed)?

HOW TO ADDRESS KIDNEY CHANNEL

Kidney Channel is on the front of the torso and is easily accessible when the practitioner sits in seiza to the side of the client's hara. Kidney may be worked bilaterally in this area, without a Mother-hand, or one side at a time with the Mother-hand in the client's hara. The channel runs up through the belly of rectus abdominis, approximately $\frac{1}{2}$ inch lateral to the midline, and continues along the edge of the sternum to finish at KI-27 in the depression below the medial end of the clavicle (Fig. 8-4).

The easiest method of accessing the Kidney Channel in the leg is with the client lying prone. The practitioner sits, the client's knee is flexed, and his foot rests on the practitioner's thigh. This makes the client's medial side of his leg more accessible. Your Mother-hand is your outside hand, and it is placed on the client's foot. Use your Son-hand to work up Kidney Channel, starting at KI-1 (in the depression just proximal to the ball of the foot), over the foot, through the loop on the ankle just behind the medial malleolus, then up through the medial head of gastrocnemius to the medial side of the popliteal fossa, where the

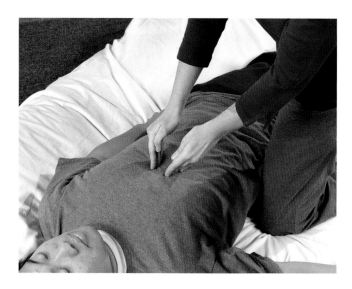

FIGURE 8-4 ■ Kidney Channel being addressed in the torso.

tendons of semimembranosus and semitendino-
sus meet. To work the upper leg, move to a lunge
facing the client's head. Your inside knee is aligned
with the client's midline, and your outside foot is
lateral to the client's hip and leg. Switch your
Mother-hand to your inside hand and rest it on
the client's sacrum. Your outside hand is now your
Son-hand. With your Son-hand, work Kidney
Channel along the medial surface of the upper leg,
just posterior to the adductors. Stop just before
you reach his inguinal region (Fig. 8-5).

HOW TO ADDRESS URINARY BLADDER CHANNEL

Urinary Bladder Channel is mostly addressed
with the client prone, with the exception of his
head and neck. To work each of the two lines of
Urinary Bladder down the back, the practitioner
is in a lunge above the client's head, with one leg
near the client's side. The channels may be worked
bilaterally in this way. If you are considerably
shorter than the client, working one side at a time
may be preferable because maintaining the proper
angle of pressure for his lower back area may be
difficult. If you decide to work one side at a time,
this may be done from the side of the client's
body, with your hara facing the channel. The
Mother-hand may be placed on the client's scapula
or sacrum. The medial Urinary Bladder Channel
runs along the lamina groove, just lateral to the
spinous processes of the vertebrae. The lateral

Urinary Bladder Channel is along the outside
edge of the erector spinae group, approximately 2
inches lateral to the midline (Fig. 8-6).

The working position for the leg is with the
client's leg straight and the ankle propped with a
pillow for knee comfort. Your Mother-hand is
placed on the client's sacrum when working the
thigh and moves to just above the knee when
working the lower leg and foot. Work either the
medial or lateral branch first. The medial branch
zigzags through the sacrum, then travels laterally
through the gluteals to the center of the transverse
gluteal fold. Follow it as it descends through the
center of the posterior thigh. It veers laterally for
the last third of the posterior thigh to the lateral
side of the popliteal fossa, then goes to the center
of the popliteal fossa to UB-40. The lateral back
branch continues from the lowest sacral foramina
along the lateral curve of the gluteal muscles. It
angles slightly medially and crosses the other posterior thigh branch of the channel about a hand's
width superior to the popliteal fossa and descends
inferiorly to UB-40. Continue to work Urinary
Bladder as it descends distally down the middle
of gastrocnemius and travels laterally to pass
between the Achilles tendon and the lateral malleolus. Follow it as it curves around the lateral
malleolus then travels along the lateral edge of the
foot to end at UB-67, on the lateral side of the
little toe's toenail (Fig. 8-7).

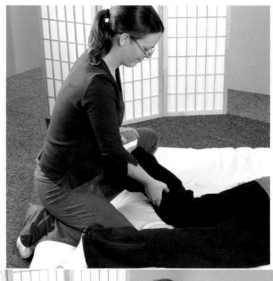

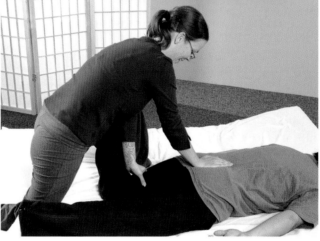

FIGURE 8-5 ■ Kidney Channel being addressed in the leg.

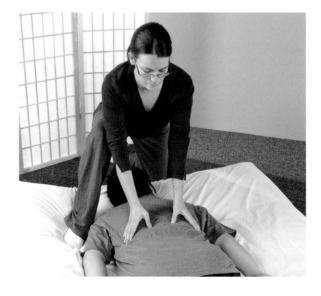

FIGURE 8-6 ■ Urinary Bladder Channel being addressed in the back.

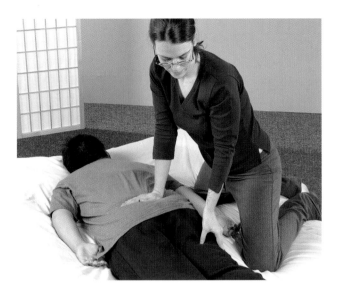

FIGURE 8-7   ■   Urinary Bladder Channel being addressed in the leg.

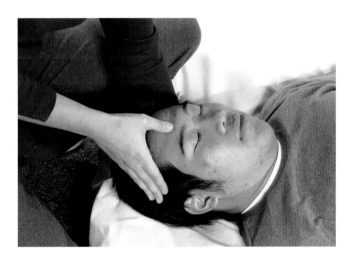

FIGURE 8-8   ■   Urinary Bladder Channel being addressed unilaterally in the head.

To work Urinary Bladder Channel in the client's head and neck, the client is supine. This part of the channel may be worked unilaterally or bilaterally, without a Mother-hand. Sit in seiza at the client's head. With your thumbs or fingers, work from UB-1 at the inside corner of the client's eye, up the forehead, over the crown, and down the back of his head to the base of his occiput. For the neck, move so that you are on your knees and elbows with the back of your hands resting on the floor. With your middle fingertips, press upward into Urinary Bladder as it travels from the base of the client's occiput, down his neck, and into his lamina groove (Fig. 8-8).

CLIENT SELF-CARE FOR WATER IMBALANCE

- Take a bath, especially with Epsom salts.
- Write in a journal.
- Meditate.
- Avoid caffeine and other stimulants.
- Spend time near bodies of water, such as the ocean or a lake.

WOOD ELEMENT: LIVER AND GALLBLADDER

8-3

The Wood element represents the new life of springtime; in the body Wood is responsible for action, expression of self, and the smooth flow of Ki. The Liver functions as a detoxifier in the body, and the Gallbladder assists by storing bile. The Liver is also seen as a reservoir for the Blood and therefore is responsible for releasing it to other body tissues. The eyes are connected to Wood and bring vision to the processes of planning and decision making, which relate to Liver and Gallbladder, respectively. The tendons are the body tissue of Wood and give the body its flexibility and the capacity to "bend with the wind."

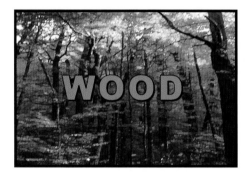

SYMPTOMS OF WOOD ELEMENT IMBALANCE

When Wood is out of balance, the liver and gallbladder organs may have disorders, and detoxification of the body may be compromised. Even if the gallbladder has been removed, the Gallbladder Channel is still present and should be addressed. Vision problems and eye problems relate to the Wood element, such as blurred vision or dry or painful eyes. In women the Liver relates to certain aspects of the menstrual cycle, and a Liver imbalance may be noted by scanty or no menstruation. Tendon issues such as repetitive motion injuries may occur with a Wood disharmony, and a lack of flexibility or stiffness in the muscles may also be present. Because the Gallbladder Channel is on the sides of the body, the right and left sides of the body may look different in the case of a Wood imbalance. Pain may exist in the neck and shoulders, the sides of the body, or the hips. Migraine headaches are often associated with a Wood imbal-

ance because they usually affect only one side of the head and/or vision.

The Wood element governs the smooth flow of Ki, including the emotions. The Wood element is particularly affected by the repression of any emotions. Anger is the emotion of Wood, and it can be especially toxic when held in and not expressed. When Wood is out of balance the person may seem to get angry quite easily or may never be able to get angry at all.

Because the Wood element is associated with self-expression, assertiveness is a key aspect of healthy Wood. A person who is timid and shy is not able to engage in self-expression. Someone who is overly assertive, to the point of being aggressive, is out of balance to the other extreme. Negative habits such as overeating, drinking, or using drugs commonly develop when people are unable to express themselves freely.

Flexibility of the mind can also be affected by a Wood imbalance. When a person is mentally stiff, clarity can be affected. He or she may have difficulty creating effective plans and decisions for the long term (Liver Channel effect) or short term (Gallbladder Channel effect). Too much planning or the inability to make plans can lead to no action being taken at all.

ASSESSMENT QUESTIONS

- How flexible are you?
- Do you have any tendon or joint injuries?
- Do you have any liver or gallbladder disorders?
- Do you tend to express yourself readily?
- How do you respond when something angers you?
- How do you feel about decision making and planning?
- Do you crave sour foods (e.g., citrus, vinegar)?

HOW TO ADDRESS LIVER CHANNEL

Liver Channel may be worked in the torso from the side of the client's hara, with the practitioner sitting in seiza. Your Mother-hand is on the client's hara. From about an inch superior to his pubic bone, your Son-hand follows the channel as it angles laterally and superiorly to LV-13,

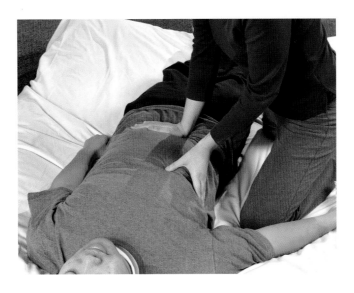

FIGURE 8-9 ■ Liver Channel being addressed in the torso.

which is just inferior to the tip of his eleventh rib (floating rib). Continue to angle superiorly and medially to end on LV-14, which is on the mammary line between ribs 6 and 7 (Fig. 8-9).

The working position for Liver Channel in the leg is with the client supine and his leg flexed in a figure 4 position. The client's heel should be above his opposite knee if comfortable, and the knee of the leg to be worked is out to the side. The client may need propping under the knee, either with a small pillow or on your thigh, if his leg is not very flexible. With your hara facing the client's knee and your Mother-hand on the client's hara, your Son-hand works up Liver Channel in his leg. With your Son-hand, start on the lateral corner of the client's big toe, travel up between his first and second metatarsal bones, then follow the channel up the edge of his tibia. Approximately two thirds of the way up the client's leg, Liver Channel swoops posteriorly to his knee, then travels posterior to his gracilis into his inguinal area. Stop working just before you reach the client's inguinal area (Fig. 8-10).

HOW TO ADDRESS GALLBLADDER CHANNEL

Gallbladder Channel is best addressed with the client in side-lying position. His neck and head may be accessed by the practitioner sitting in seiza while facing the same direction as the top of the client's head, holding his shoulder with the Mother-hand. Your Son-hand works from GB-1, at the outside corner of the client's eye, and follows the channel to his ear and then along the zigzag across the side of his head to GB-20 at the edge of his occiput. From there it travels to GB-21 on the top of the client's shoulder.

Gallbladder channel in the client's torso may be addressed with the practitioner in a lunge and her Mother-hand at the client's hip or shoulder. On the side of the body, the Gallbladder Channel zigzags back and forth a few times. Follow the channel as it reemerges below the axilla and angles inferiorly and medially to the eighth rib then travels almost straight posteriorly to the tip of the twelfth rib. From there, GB again travels anteriorly along the anterior iliac crest to the anterior superior iliac spine. From the anterior superior iliac spine, GB travels posteriorly to GB-30, located one third of the way between the greater trochanter and the sacrum. GB then angles anteriorly to descend the upper lateral leg along the iliotibial tract and the fibula in the lower lateral leg. Approximately one third of the way down the fibula, GB travels anteriorly in a straight line approximately 1 inch to GB-36, then angles inferiorly back to the fibula and on the foot catches the lateral tendon of the fourth toe. GB ends at GB-44, on the lateral side of the corner of the

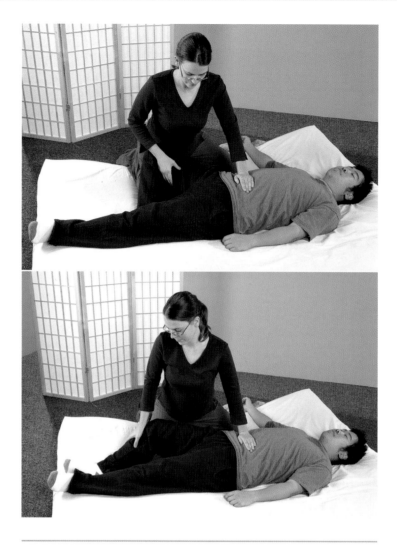

FIGURE 8-10 ■ Liver Channel being addressed in the leg.

fourth toe's nail. The client's leg and foot also may be addressed in a lunge position, with your leg across the client's lower legs and your Mother-hand at his hip (Fig. 8-11).

CLIENT SELF-CARE FOR WOOD IMBALANCE

- Spend time in nature, particularly in the woods.
- Write down a goal and plans to achieve that goal.
- Exercise regularly.
- Find healthy ways to express anger (e.g., pounding a pillow).
- Avoid excesses (e.g., food, drink, exercise).

FIRE ELEMENT: HEART, SMALL INTESTINE, HEART PROTECTOR, AND TRIPLE HEATER

The Fire element represents the excitement and heat of summertime and the spirit or conscious-ness of the body. The Heart, which houses the Shen, is considered the emperor, and is protected and assisted by Small Intestine and Heart Protec-tor. Small Intestine is responsible for assimilation, and Triple Heater controls circulation throughout the body. The body tissue of Fire is the blood vessels.

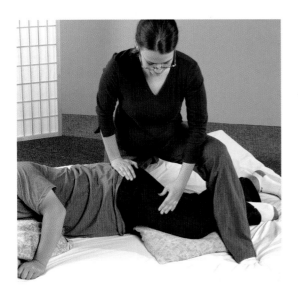

FIGURE 8-11 ▦ Gallbladder Channel being addressed in side-lying position.

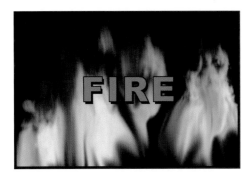

SYMPTOMS OF FIRE ELEMENT IMBALANCE

When Fire is out of balance, obvious symptoms may include problems with the heart organ or the small intestine. Blood pressure issues, atherosclerosis, and other circulatory disorders may be present. The person may have difficulty with temperature regulation, often feel too warm or too cold, or have cold hands and feet, or sweat excessively. Triple Heater in its circulatory function also relates to the lymphatic system, and an imbalance may lead the person to be prone to edema. Triple Heater also circulates the Wei Qi, or Defensive Qi, and is therefore connected to the immune system. Someone who often gets sick or has many allergies may have a Triple Heater disharmony. Small Intestine is said to separate the pure from the impure and therefore has an important role in the digestive process. If a person has difficulty

assimilating nutrients, Small Intestine may be out of balance. Heart is connected to the tongue, and through this, speech; as such, Fire is associated with communication. Speech impediments such as stuttering may indicate a Heart imbalance.

The condition of the Heart is easily seen in a person's complexion. It should have a healthy pinkness, and the eyes should be bright and expressive. If the face is overly red or too pale, a Fire imbalance may be present. The emotion for Fire is joy or contentment. If someone is always laughing or giggling, especially at inappropriate times, this indicates a Fire disharmony. Likewise, a Fire imbalance also may be present if a person almost never laughs.

Several conditions are related to an imbalance in the Shen, which resides in the Heart. If the Shen is scattered, the person's spirit is not present in the body. This can be a result of shock or coma, but schizophrenia is also considered scattered Shen. Many mental illnesses are related to disorders of the Shen. The Shen is also associated with epilepsy. Insomnia is sometimes linked to the Shen being unable to rest in the Heart for the night.

Small Intestine controls assimilation, which applies to concepts and emotions as well as nutrients and other substances. To learn something new or process an event that has taken place, a person must assimilate it into his or her being. Part of that experience must become that person; in other words, he or she must own it. Small Intestine is often related to when a person experiences symptoms long after a traumatic event. A person may be unable to assimilate an experience at the time it occurred because of being in shock. Also, if a person is able to take in new information but unable to remember it clearly or put it to use, Small Intestine may need addressing.

Fire relates to connection, both with the self and others. The connection to self is most closely associated with the Heart and the Shen. Heart and Small Intestine connect the Shen and the Ki, linking the spirit with the physical processes of the body. Heart Protector and Triple Heater connect the person to others and create emotional boundaries. If a Fire imbalance is present a person may have few trusted, close friends because of excessive emotional barriers. The opposite may

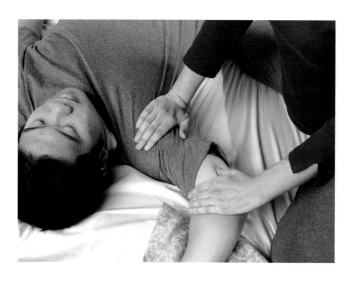

FIGURE 8-12 ■ Heart Channel being addressed in supine position.

also be true, as with people who wear their hearts on their sleeves.

ASSESSMENT QUESTIONS

- How is your circulation?
- Do you have any heart conditions or blood pressure problems?
- Do you assimilate nutrition easily?
- Do you assimilate new information easily?
- Do you get sick often?
- Do you crave bitter foods or drinks (e.g., coffee, chocolate, alcohol)?

HOW TO ADDRESS HEART CHANNEL

The working position for Heart is with the client supine and his arm up by the side of his head. If needed, a pillow may be used to prop the elbow. Sit facing Heart Channel, with one knee near the client's axilla and the other near his hand. Your Mother-hand is placed near the client's axilla, and your Son-hand works along the channel toward his hand. Heart begins in the center of the client's axilla and travels along the anterior (Yin) aspect of his arm. In the client's upper arm, the channel is between his biceps brachii and triceps brachii, and in his forearm it travels along the medial aspect of his ulna. Heart crosses the edge of the client's palm to end on HT-9, on the radial side of the corner of the little finger's nail (Fig. 8-12).

HOW TO ADDRESS SMALL INTESTINE CHANNEL

Small Intestine Channel in the client's neck and head is addressed with the practitioner sitting in seiza above the client's head. Your Mother-hand supports his slightly turned head. Your Son-hand works the channel from the superior angle of the client's scapula to diagonally across his neck, crossing sternocleidomastoid and the mandible, onto the client's face to just below his cheekbone, and then traveling to SI-19 just in front of the tragus of his ear (Fig. 8-13).

The easiest way to access Small Intestine in the scapular region is with the client prone, with his arm by his side, palms facing down. From SI-10 in an indentation just posterior to the acromion process, follow the channel as it travels inferiorly and medially to SI-11 in the center of the client's scapula, then as it ascends directly superior to SI-12 in the middle of supraspinatus. SI then travels medially (and slightly inferiorly) to SI-13 and from there it runs superiorly to C7. Your Mother-hand may be on the client's shoulder or back while working this section (Fig. 8-14).

You can rest the client's hand on your thigh and work from SI-1 through his little finger, his medial wrist, and up the channel in his arm along the medial edge of the ulna. When you reach his elbow you can place his arm in the working position for Small Intestine; flex it and place his hand on his opposite shoulder. Use your Mother-hand to hold the client's elbow as you continue

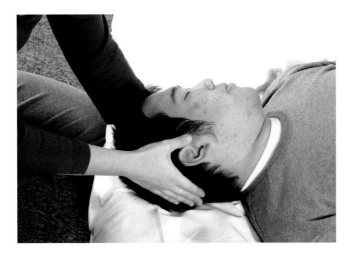

FIGURE 8-13 ■ Small Intestine Channel being addressed in the neck and head.

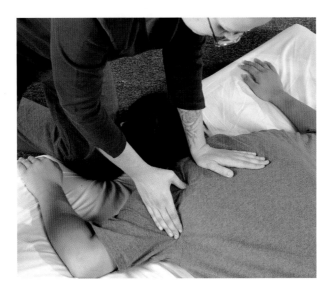

FIGURE 8-14 ■ Small Intestine Channel being addressed in prone position.

thumbing between the olecranon process and the medial epicondyle of the humerus and through the center of triceps brachii and the axillary crease to SI-10 (Fig. 8-15).

HOW TO ADDRESS HEART PROTECTOR CHANNEL

The working position for Heart Protector Channel is with the client's arm at a 90-degree angle from his body with his palm up. Your Mother-hand is on the client's shoulder. HP starts at HP-1, which is found in his fourth intercostal space, just lateral and slightly superior to his nipple and travels superiorly to his axilla. Follow it through the client's anterior axilla, between the heads of his biceps brachii, then through the center of his elbow. From there the channel travels between flexor carpi radialis and palmaris longus and through the center of his palm to end at HP-9, on the radial side of the tip of his middle finger (Fig. 8-16).

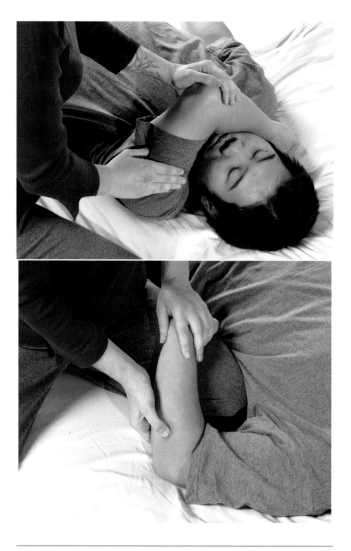

FIGURE 8-15 ■ Small Intestine Channel being addressed in the arm in supine position.

HOW TO ADDRESS TRIPLE HEATER CHANNEL

Triple Heater Channel in the client's neck and head is addressed with the practitioner sitting in seiza above his head. Your Mother-hand supports his head, which is slightly turned, and your Son-hand works from TH-14 at the client's acromion process medially along supraspinatus, then moves up the lateral border of trapezius to his occiput. From the most lateral edge of the occiput, TH branches anteriorly toward the face under the earlobe. It circles laterally around the earlobe to where the earlobe attaches to the head, then rises superiorly to TH-22 on the most lateral aspect of the zygomatic arch. TH crosses in a straight line to end at TH-23 on the lateral end of the eyebrow (Fig. 8-17).

To work Triple Heater Channel in the client's arm, support it on your thigh and while your Mother-hand holds his hand. Your Son-hand starts TH-1 on the ulnar side of the corner of the fourth finger's nail. It travels along the fourth finger's tendon and up the posterior forearm just to the medial side of the midline. The client's arm is repositioned at this point to allow for proper body mechanics. The client's elbow is flexed and his hand is placed on his opposite shoulder. Your Son-hand works Triple Heater Channel through his olecranon process, up through the center of the lateral head of triceps brachii, and through

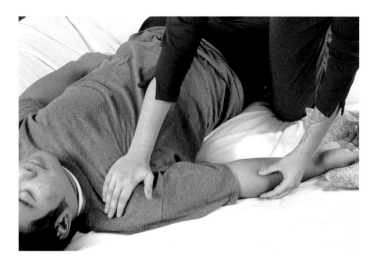

FIGURE 8-16 ▦ Heart Protector Channel being addressed in the arm in supine position.

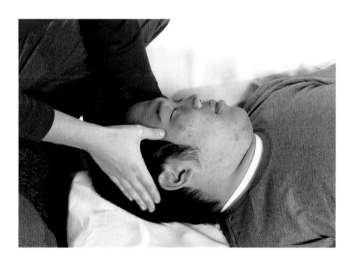

FIGURE 8-17 ▦ Triple Heater Channel being addressed in the head.

posterior deltoid to the acromion process. TH then travels medially along the supraspinatus (Fig. 8-18).

CLIENT SELF-CARE FOR FIRE IMBALANCE

- Have a long conversation with a good friend.
- Watch a funny movie and laugh out loud.
- Meditate.
- Go to a party.
- Avoid caffeine and other stimulants.

EARTH ELEMENT: SPLEEN AND STOMACH

The Earth element relates to nourishment, centeredness, and transformation. Stomach takes in food, and Spleen transforms the purest part of the food into Ki. Earth is associated with the mouth, through which a person nourishes the body, and the fleshy parts of the muscles. Earth is the season of change, the transitions between each of the seasons, and is related to stability through transitions in a person's life.

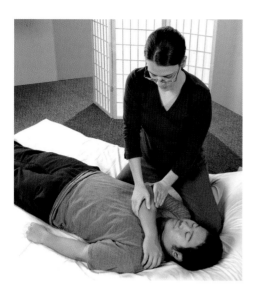

FIGURE 8-18 ■ Triple Heater Channel being addressed in the upper arm in supine position.

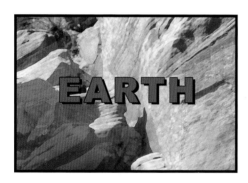

SYMPTOMS OF EARTH ELEMENT IMBALANCE

The physical manifestations of an Earth imbalance may include any sort of digestive disorder, such as acid reflux, bloating, or loose stools. A person may have a loss of appetite or pain in the abdomen. If Spleen is not transforming the food into Ki, fatigue will result, and women may have symptoms such as scanty menstruation or dizziness. The female reproductive hormones are connected with the Earth element, and issues with fertility are considered an Earth imbalance. When Earth is out of balance, the flesh may be achy and the person may not want to exercise.

Spleen provides the sense of taste and the enjoyment of food; when it is out of balance various eating disorders may occur. A person may overeat, want to eat all the time, eat too quickly, or have no appetite. The flavor for the Earth element is sweet; craving sweets or eating a lot of sweet things indicates an Earth imbalance.

Spleen is also said to house thought and is responsible for processing new ideas as well as food. If a person thinks too much or constantly worries, the appetite is affected because Spleen cannot keep up. When a person eats while obsessively worrying, digestion often is poor.

Stomach, which accepts food, is responsible for all aspects of acceptance in life. If a person has difficulty accepting nourishment in the form of emotional support from others, the Earth element is involved. Eating disorders are often related to the inability to accept nourishment on other levels. Also, Stomach is located at the front of the body and is related to the "front" that a person puts out to others. When an Earth imbalance is present, often this front is overly nurturing toward others or tries to please everyone else.

ASSESSMENT QUESTIONS

- How is your digestion?
- How is your menstrual cycle (for women)?
- What are your eating habits like?
- Do you crave sweet foods?
- Do you tend to overthink or worry too much?
- Do you exercise regularly?

HOW TO ADDRESS SPLEEN CHANNEL

Spleen Channel in the torso is worked with the practitioner sitting in seiza next to the client's hara. Spleen travels up the belly 1 inch lateral to the edge of the client's rectus abdominis angling out at his ribcage to continue ascending ½ inch lateral to his nipple to SP-20, which is approximately 1 inch inferior and slightly medial to LU-1. Do not work through breast tissue; skip over that part of the channel. Continue down the side of the client's ribcage to end at SP-21, approximately one hand's width inferior to his axilla and in line with the center of the his axilla. Your Mother-hand may be placed on the client's hara to work this section (Fig. 8-19).

The working position for Spleen in the leg is with the client's leg slightly flexed in a figure 4 position. The client's knee points outward, and his foot faces his opposite ankle. A pillow may be

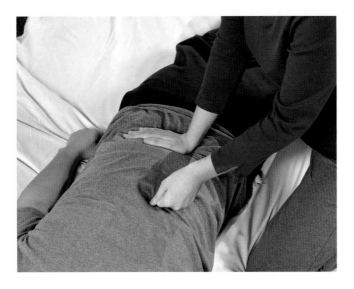

FIGURE 8-19 ■ Spleen Channel being addressed in the torso.

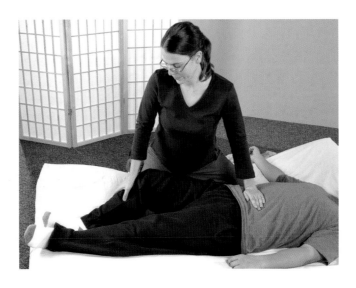

FIGURE 8-20 ■ Spleen Channel being addressed in the leg in supine position.

needed to prop the client's knee, depending on his flexibility. With your Mother-hand in the client's hara, face Spleen Channel with a wide stance. Use your Son-hand to work the channel from SP-1 on the medial aspect of the corner of the big toe's nail, through the medial edge of his foot, and anterior to the medial malleolus. Follow the channel along the calf just anterior to gastrocnemius (hook in toward the tibia with your thumb), past the medial border of the patella then between vastus medialis and rectus femoris. Stop just before you reach the client's inguinal area (Fig. 8-20).

HOW TO ADDRESS STOMACH CHANNEL

Stomach Channel in the torso may be worked with the practitioner sitting in seiza next to the client's hara. The channel flows from the midpoint of the clavicle down along the nipple line. At the level of the fifth rib, it angles gently toward the

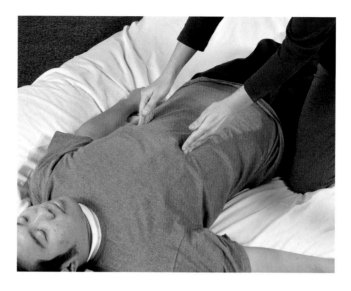

FIGURE 8-21 ■ Stomach Channel being addressed bilaterally in the torso.

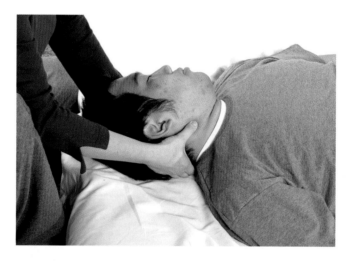

FIGURE 8-22 ■ Stomach Channel being addressed in the neck.

lateral edge of the rectus abdominis. The channel may be worked bilaterally in his torso, or one side at a time, using your Mother-hand in his hara (Fig. 8-21).

To work Stomach in the client's neck and head, the practitioner sits in seiza above his head. Your Mother-hand supports the client's head, and your Son-hand works carefully from just under his eye in line with his pupil (ST-1, ST-2, and ST-3) down to just past the corner of the mouth. It angles laterally to the jawline, then travels posteriorly along the mandible to ST-6 in the center of the masseter. From there a branch ascends directly up to the superior edge of temporalis. The channel continues inferiorly along either side of the esophagus then descends toward the head of the clavicle where it runs horizontally along the superior edge of the clavicle to the midpoint (Fig. 8-22).

The working position for Stomach in the leg is with the client's leg straight and his toes pointing toward the ceiling. Propping may be necessary to keep the client's leg from rolling laterally. Stomach Channel travels along the client's lateral

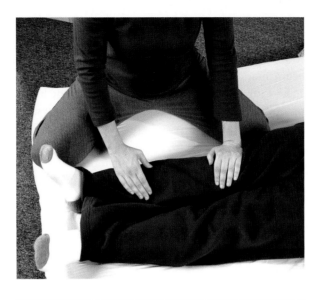

FIGURE 8-23 ■ Stomach Channel being addressed in the leg.

edge of rectus femoris, the lateral border of the patella, and tibialis anterior. It continues along the lateral edge of his tibia in his lower leg. A slight jog laterally occurs about halfway down the client's lower leg for the point ST-40. Stomach Channel flows along the lateral edge of the tendon of the second toe and follows it distally to end at ST-45, on the lateral end of the toenail. Your Mother-hand is in the client's hara while working his thigh and may be moved down to just above his knee to work the channel in his lower leg and foot (Fig. 8-23).

SELF-CARE FOR EARTH IMBALANCE

- Get regular exercise.
- Do something nice for yourself.
- Cook a healthy meal and enjoy each bite.
- Sing.
- Avoid sweet foods and cold or frozen foods.

The best and most beautiful things in the world cannot be seen or even touched. They must be felt with the heart.
~Helen Keller

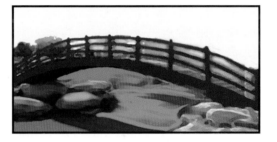

DOCUMENTING SHIATSU TREATMENT SESSIONS

It is important for the shiatsu practitioner to document client treatment sessions. This documentation, also called charting, is a record of the treatments the practitioner has performed on the client. Documentation of each treatment should include the client's name, the client's age, results of the pretreatment interview with the client, the jitsu channel and the kyo channel from the hara assessment, results from all the other assessments that the practitioner performed on the client, the channels the practitioner addressed and the techniques used on those channels, the manner in which the practitioner addressed other areas of kyo and jitsu on the client, any other techniques the practitioner used during the session, the client's response to the techniques used, pertinent information from the posttreatment discussion, and recommendations the practitioner gave the client for self-care. The documentation should be kept together with the intake form (also known as a pretreatment form or health history form) the client has filled out. Because of the confidential nature of this client information, it needs to be kept in a private and secure location, such as a locked filing cabinet.

Besides being required by law in some states and municipalities, this detailed log of information is a valuable tool for the practitioner. It can be used for planning treatment sessions because the practitioner can determine what techniques and suggestions for self-care have been helpful and useful for the client and which ones have not. The practitioner can note progress the client has made with his or her health issues. Also, if there are questions about what was said and done during a particular treatment, the practitioner has a written record and does not have to rely on his or her memory.

Shiatsu practitioners should research the laws regarding treatment documentation requirements in the cities and states in which they practice and make sure they are in compliance with these laws.

1. The only way for you to become better at shiatsu is to practice as many treatments on as many different people as you can. Practice on at least two clients a week. These practice sessions should be documented. The following is a list of important information to include when charting the treatment session. You may notice that it is a culmination of previous chapter workbook activities. These served as building blocks for comprehensive treatment session documentation.

   - Client's name
   - Client's age
   - Results of the pretreatment interview with the client
   - What channel was jitsu and what channel was kyo in the hara assessment

   - Results from all the other assessments you performed
   - Incorporation of specific channel work into the treatment—what channels you addressed and the techniques you used on those channels
   - How you addressed other areas of kyo and jitsu on the client
   - Any other techniques you used
   - How the client responded to the techniques you used
   - Pertinent information from the posttreatment discussion
   - Recommendations you gave the client for self-care

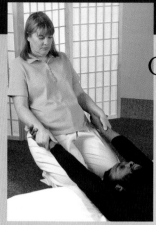

ADDITIONAL TECHNIQUES

OBJECTIVES

Upon completion of this chapter, the reader will have the information necessary to do the following:
1. Perform additional shiatsu techniques in side position and for the hara, anterior legs, anterior arms, neck, face, back, and posterior legs.
2. Perform shiatsu treatments in a personal, creative style.
3. Document the treatment session.

T he beauty and grace, as well as the fun, of shiatsu include the continual incorporation of new techniques. Shiatsu has never been a static form of bodywork. Its origins are traditional and modern, tried and true, simple and complex. When the shiatsu practitioner has mastered the Basic Kata, and has a good grasp of techniques to address typical element imbalances, it is time to experiment with new methods.

What follows are suggestions for additional techniques for the shiatsu practitioner to use. Every practitioner is encouraged to take continuing education classes in shiatsu, trade ideas with other practitioners, attend conventions to interact with many different practitioners, and take every opportunity available to learn more. All these are chances for the shiatsu practitioner to grow and to stretch. Shiatsu is a living art form. If your style becomes stagnant, you may not be able to offer the best to your clients.

These techniques are not intended as a protocol. That is, they are not necessarily meant to be performed in the order in which they are presented. Instead, try interspersing these techniques throughout your treatment, whenever and wherever they would be particularly useful. Most of all, have fun. Enjoy the movements and enjoy the practice of shiatsu.

Ampuku   Barefoot Shiatu   Kenbiki

HARA

9-1 **KENBIKI**

Kenbiki is an Anma technique designed to release muscular tension. It involves the practitioner using both hands to rock and jostle either specific regions in the body or the client's entire body.

The Wave

Sit in seiza (or come up on one knee, depending on the size of your client) perpendicular to the client. In a fluid motion, push the lateral side of his hara that is closest to you away with both hands, then pull the lateral side of his hara furthest from you toward you with both hands. Repeat several times, traveling up and down the client's hara as you do so (Fig. 9-1, *A* and *B*).

Stomach Channel Jostle

Sit in seiza (or come up on one knee, depending on the size of your client) perpendicular to the client. Hold on to his Stomach Channel with both hands and jostle his hara. Repeat several times, traveling up and down the client's hara as you do so (Fig. 9-1, *C*).

Trunk Sway

Kneel (or come up on one knee, depending on the size of your client) next to the client, facing his head. Using dragon's mouth, hold the lateral sides of his trunk just under the ribs and sway his body, working down his torso (Fig. 9-1, *D*).

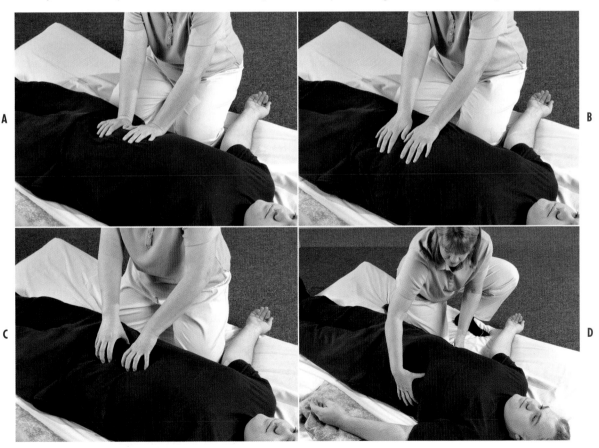

FIGURE 9-1 ■ Kenbiki. **A** and **B,** The wave. **C,** Stomach channel jostle. **D,** Trunk sway.

AMPUKU

Ampuku is deep palming and massaging in the client's hara. Kneel (or come up on one knee, depending on the size of your client) perpendicular to him. With both your hands, palm deeply around the client's hara (Fig. 9-2).

ANTERIOR LEGS

LIVER CHANNEL

To work Liver Channel in the client's upper leg, get into a lunge position. Flex the client's knee and hip and rotate her leg laterally. The client's knee is resting on your thigh and her shin is resting in your hara. Rest your outside hand as a Mother-hand on the client's knee. Use your inside forearm on her Liver Channel (Fig. 9-3, *A*).

To work Liver Channel in the client's lower leg, move to seiza and rest her lower leg in your lap. Palm, then use your thumb, fingers, forearm, and elbow on her Liver Channel (Fig. 9-3, *B*).

Put the client's leg in a figure 4 position. With your hara facing her upper leg, place a Mother-hand on the client's opposite anterior superior iliac spine and support under her lateral knee with your other hand. Use your inside knee on the client's Liver Channel (Fig. 9-3, *C*).

To work Liver Channel from across the client's body, put her in the Liver stretch (working)

position. Place a small pillow under her knee for support. With your hara facing the client's upper leg, come up on one knee. Place your Mother-hand in her hara, then use your Son-hand to palm and thumb her Liver Channel (Fig. 9-3, *D*).

STOMACH AND SPLEEN CHANNELS

Forearm and Elbow on the Stomach and Spleen Channels

Kneel perpendicular to the client in a wide stance. Rest a Mother-hand in her hara. Use your other forearm on her Stomach and Spleen Channels (Fig. 9-4, *A*).

Use your elbow on Stomach Channel in the client's upper leg (Fig. 9-4, *B*).

Sit back and rest the client's lower leg on your thighs. Rest a Mother-hand on her knee and use the elbow of your other arm on Spleen Channel in the client's lower leg (Fig. 9-4, *C*).

Earth Makka-Ho Stretch

Kneel perpendicular to the client's leg. With one hand on her ankle and the other hand on her knee, flex her knee and swing her lower leg into the Earth Makka-Ho position. Rest a hand on the client's knee as a Mother-hand and palm and thumb her Stomach Channel (Fig. 9-4, *D*).

⚠ **This technique should only be performed on clients who are flexible enough to receive it**

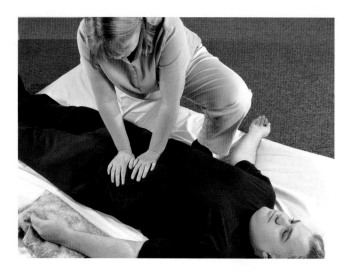

FIGURE 9-2 ■ Ampuku.

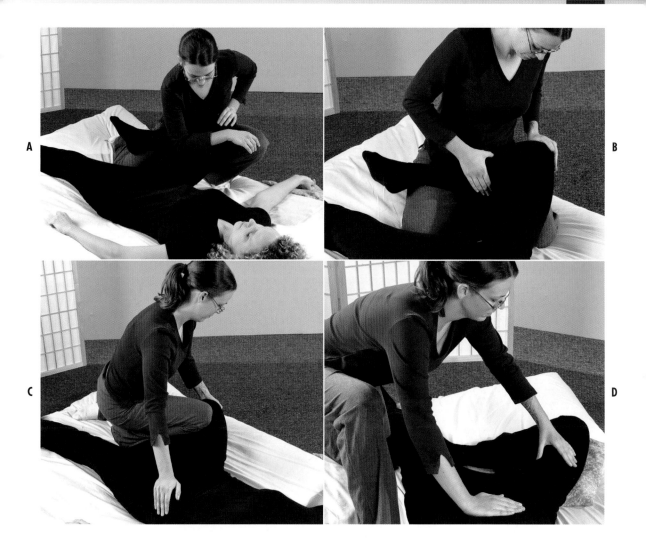

FIGURE 9-3 ■ **A,** Forearm on Liver Channel in upper leg. **B,** Working Liver Channel in lower leg. **C,** Knee on Liver Channel. **D,** Working Liver Channel from across the body.

and who do not have knee joint or hip joint issues.

Barefoot Shiatsu

Stand perpendicular to the client's leg. Place a small pillow under her knee. Use the soles of your feet and your toes on her Stomach and Spleen Channels (Fig. 9-4, *E*).

9-4 ANTERIOR ARMS

FULL-LENGTH ARM STRETCH

Lay the client's arm out at a 90-degree angle from his body. Sit in seiza (or come up on one knee, depending on the size of the client) with your hara facing his arm. With one hand on the client's shoulder and the other on the client's wrist, lean forward to give his arm a full-length arm stretch (Fig. 9-5, *A*).

FOREARM ON CLIENT'S ARM AND FOREARM CHANNELS

Lay the client's arm out at a 90-degree angle from his body. Sit in seiza (or come up on one knee, depending on the size of the client) with your hara facing the client's arm. With your inside forearm on his shoulder joint, use your other forearm down the length of his arm and forearm (Fig. 9-5, *B*).

Text continued on p. 206

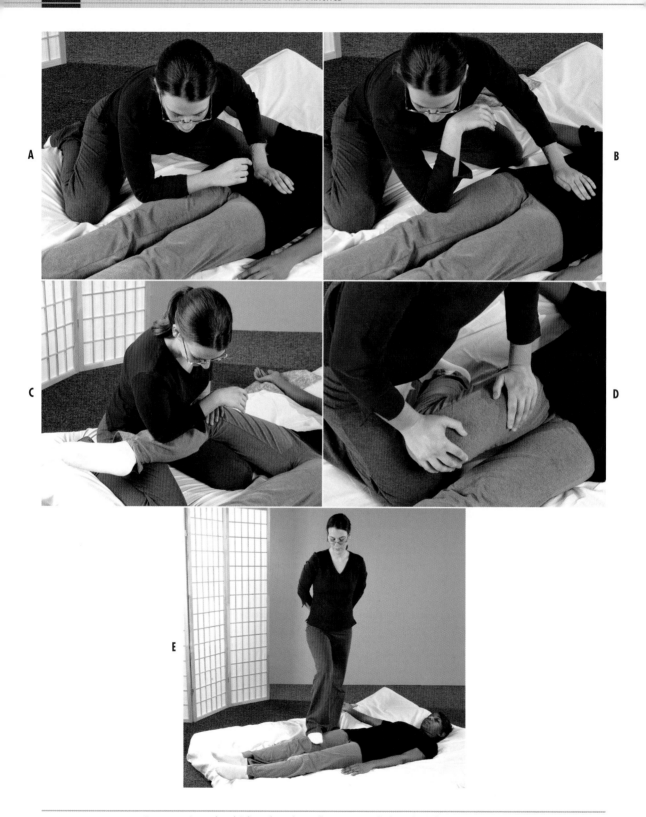

FIGURE 9-4 ■ **A,** Forearm on Stomach and Spleen Channels. **B,** Elbow on Stomach Channel. **C,** Elbow on Spleen Channel. **D,** Working Stomach Channel in Earth Makka-Ho. **E,** Barefoot shiatsu on Stomach and Spleen Channels.

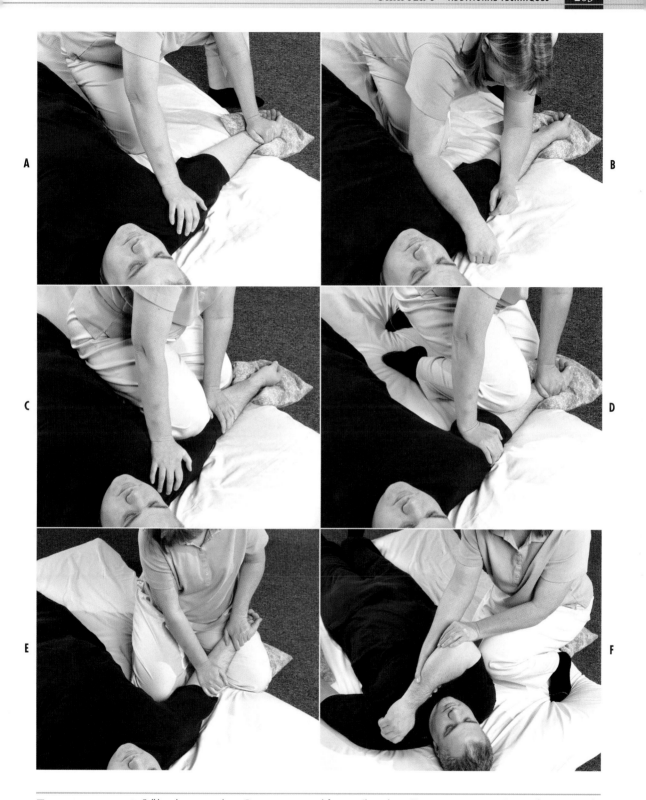

FIGURE 9-5 ■ **A,** Full-length arm stretch. **B,** Forearm on arm and forearm Channels. **C,** Knee on upper arm. **D,** Knee on forearm. **E,** Palm press into arm. **F,** Knee on Triple Heater Channel in upper arm.

Continued

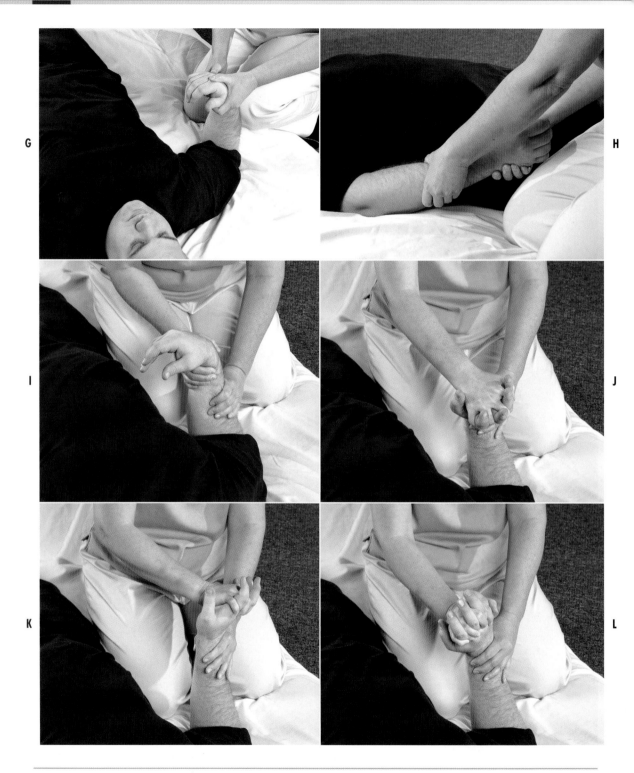

FIGURE 9-5, cont'd ■ **G,** Knee on forearm. **H,** Radial and ulnar press. **I,** Milking the forearm. **J-L,** Range of motion on the wrist.

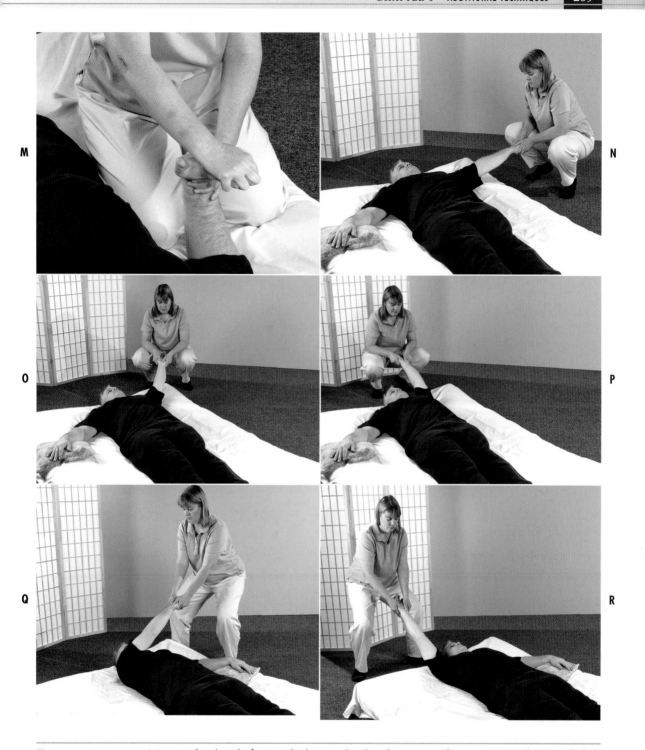

FIGURE 9-5, cont'd ■ **M,** Stretching the fingers and palm. **N-P,** Stretching the arm out in three positions. **Q** and **R,** Cross the body stretch and range of motion of the arm.

Continued

S

T

U

FIGURE 9-5, cont'd ▪ **S-U,** Cross the body stretch and range of motion of the arm.

KNEE ON CLIENT'S ARM AND FOREARM CHANNELS

Lay the client's arm out at a 90-degree angle from his body. With your Mother-hand on the client's shoulder joint and your other hand just distal to his elbow joint, use your knee on his upper arm (Fig. 9-5, *C*).

When you have nearly reached the client's elbow joint, move your Mother-hand to just proximal to his elbow joint and your other hand down to your client's wrist. Use your knee on his forearm (Fig. 9-5, *D*).

PALM PRESS INTO ARM

Lay the client's arm out at a 90-degree angle from his body. Sit in seiza with your hara facing the client's arm. Rest his wrist on your thigh. Hold his wrist with your outside hand. On the client's forearm, palm inward with your inside hand while pulling his arm into a press. The force is downward and toward the client's elbow (Fig. 9-5, *E*).

KNEE ON CLIENT'S TRIPLE HEATER CHANNEL

Kneel perpendicular to the client by his upper arm. Flex the client's elbow and hold his arm across his body. One of your hands holds his arm approximately halfway between his wrist and elbow; the other hand rests on his elbow. To work Triple Heater Channel in the client's upper arm, pull his arm toward your knee as you press in with your knee. A push-pull action should occur at the same time (Fig. 9-5, *F*).

Place the client's flexed elbow on the futon. Use your knee on Triple Heater Channel in the client's forearm. As you press in with your knee, pull his forearm toward your knee. A push-pull action should occur at the same time (Fig. 9-5, *G*).

RADIAL AND ULNAR PRESS

Sit in seiza, facing your client's head, at approximately a 45-degree angle from his body. With your inside hand, "shake hands" with your client. With your outside hand, alternate pressing along the radial and ulnar sides of his forearm, working your way from the elbow down to the wrist. Move the client's arm in an up-and-down wavelike motion as you press (Fig. 9-5, *H*).

MILK THE CLIENT'S FOREARM

Sit in seiza, facing your client's head, at approximately a 45-degree angle from his body. Place the client's flexed elbow on the futon. Support his wrist with your inside hand. Milk his forearm with your outside hand (Fig. 9-5, *I*).

RANGE OF MOTION ON THE CLIENT'S WRIST

Sit in seiza, facing your client's head, at approximately a 45-degree angle from his body. Stabilize the client's wrist with your outside hand. With your inside hand, interlace your fingers with his fingers and perform range of motion on his wrist several times clockwise, then several times counterclockwise (Fig. 9-5, *J-L*).

STRETCH THE CLIENT'S PALM AND FINGERS

Sit in seiza, facing your client's head, at approximately a 45-degree angle from his body. Stabilize the client's wrist with your outside hand. With your inside hand, stretch his fingers and palm toward his head (Fig. 9-5, *M*).

STRETCH THE CLIENT'S ARM

Squat perpendicular to the client and pick up his arm. Turn his arm palm side up and grasp big fish and little fish with both hands. While keeping the client's arm close to the futon, lean back for a stretch. Hold for a few seconds, then release. While holding the client's hand, move so that the client's arm is at a 45-degree angle from his head. Lean back for a stretch. Hold for a few seconds, then release. While holding the client's hand, move so that the client's arm is directly over his

head. Lean back for a stretch. Hold for a few seconds, then release (Fig. 9-5, *N-P*).

CROSS THE BODY STRETCH AND RANGE OF MOTION OF THE ARM

Stand perpendicular next to the client. Pick up the client's arm on the opposite side. Turn his arm palm side down and grasp Big Fish and Little Fish with your hands. Lean back for a stretch. Hold for a few seconds, then release. Turn the client's arm palm side up, then walk around the client while moving his arm in a range of motion. Turn the client's arm palm side down to lay it down by his body (Fig. 9-5, *Q-U*).

 9-5 # NECK

FINGERTIP PRESSES INTO THE SUBOCCIPITALS

Sit in seiza at the client's head. Cradle his occiput with both hands. Press your fingertips into his suboccipitals (Fig. 9-6, *A*).

FORWARD NECK FLEXION STRETCH

Sit in seiza at the client's head. Cross your arms and cradle his head. Perform a forward neck flexion stretch on him. Hold for a few seconds, then release (Fig. 9-6, *B*).

NECK STRETCHES WITH A SCARF

A scarf can be used to perform neck stretches. The scarf should be cotton or mostly cotton because cotton is easier to grip and feels comfortable next to the skin. It should measure approximately 30 inches long and 6 inches wide. Wider pieces of fabric folded down to 6 inches also suffice.

⚠**These stretches should not be performed on any client who has neck issues, such as arthritis or a herniated disc in the cervical region.**

Sit in seiza at the client's head. Position the scarf under his neck. Grasp the scarf as indicated in Figure 9-6, *C*. While keeping the scarf against the client's head, lean back for a posterior neck stretch. Hold for a few seconds, then release.

Turn the client's head to one side at approximately a 45-degree angle. Lean back for a

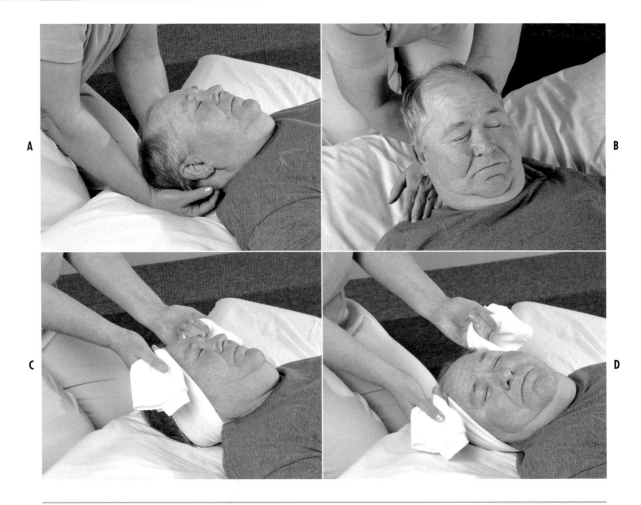

FIGURE 9-6 ■ **A,** Fingertip presses into the suboccipitals. **B,** Forward neck flexion stretch. **C,** Posterior neck stretch. **D,** Lateral neck stretch.

lateral neck stretch. Hold for a few seconds, then release. Turn his head to the other side and repeat (Fig. 9-6, *D*).

 FACE

BILATERAL PALMING OF GALLBLADDER CHANNEL

Sit in seiza at the client's head. Moderately squeeze his head and palm down his Gallbladder Channel bilaterally (Fig. 9-7, *A*).

THUMB PRESS INTO TRIPLE HEATER CHANNEL

Sit in seiza at the client's head. Use your thumb to press into Triple Heater Channel posterior to his earlobe (Fig. 9-7, *B*).

PRESS POINT OF 100 MEETINGS

Sit in seiza at the client's head. Use your thumb to press the point of 100 meetings on top of his head until you feel his Ki draw up to it (Fig. 9-7, *C*).

 BACK

KENBIKI
Sacrum

Sit in seiza (or come up on one knee, depending on the size of your client) perpendicular to the client. With both hands, jostle her sacrum (Fig. 9-8, *A*).

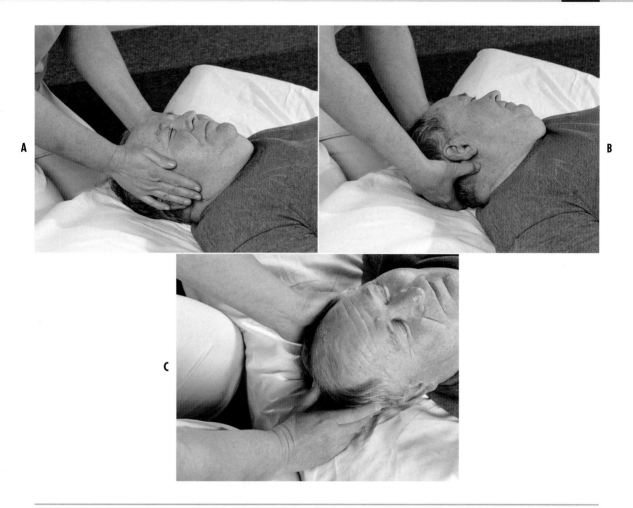

FIGURE 9-7 ■ **A,** Bilateral palming of Gallbladder Channel. **B,** Thumb press into Triple Heater Channel. **C,** Pressing point of 100 meetings.

Trunk Sway

Kneel (or come up on one knee, depending on the size of your client) next to the client, facing her head. Use dragon's mouth and hold the lateral sides of the client's trunk just under the ribs; sway her body, working down her torso (Fig. 9-8, *B*).

BAREFOOT SHIATSU

Stand perpendicular to the client. Rock his back while moving your foot up and down his back (Figure 9-8, *C*).

FOREARMS ON URINARY BLADDER CHANNEL

Kneel at the client's head. Lean forward and use your forearms and elbows on her erector spinae (Urinary Bladder channel) (Fig. 9-8, *D*).

BILATERAL THUMBING OF URINARY BLADDER CHANNEL

Kneel at the client's head and come up on one knee to thumb Urinary Bladder channel bilaterally down her back (Fig. 9-8, *E*).

 POSTERIOR LEGS

CLIENT SUPINE

Knee on the Urinary Bladder and Kidney Channels

Kneel by the client's knees, facing her head. Flex her knee and hip. Cup the client's heel with your inside hand and rest your outside hand on top of her knee. Press your inside knee along the client's Urinary Bladder and Kidney Channels in her

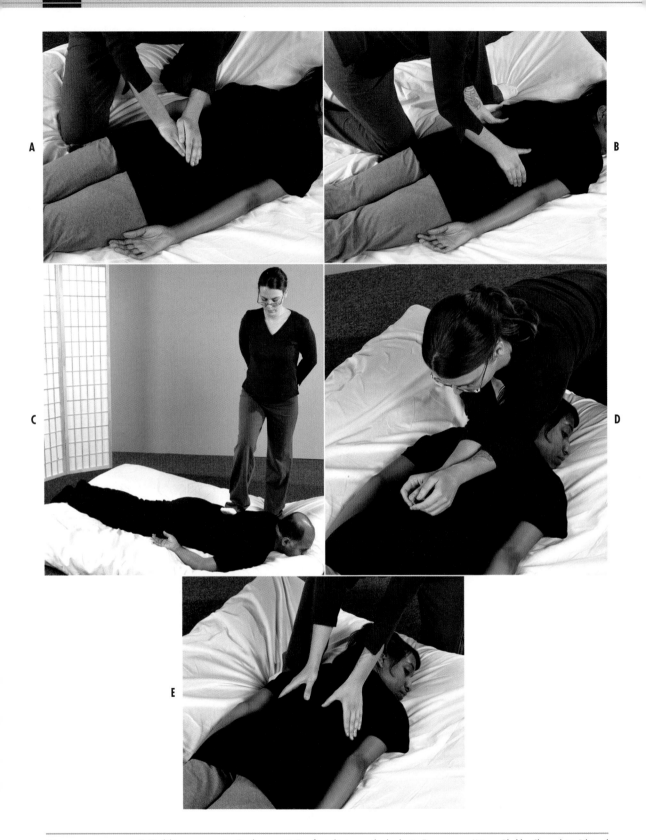

FIGURE 9-8 ■ **A,** Kenbiki on sacrum. **B,** Trunk sway. **C,** Barefoot shiatsu on the back. **D,** Forearms on Urinary Bladder Channel. **E,** Bilateral thumbing of Urinary Bladder Channel.

hamstrings from the ischial tuberosity to the popliteal fossa. While pressing in with your knee, pull the client's leg toward your knee. A push-pull action should occur at the same time (Fig. 9-9, *A* and *B*).

When your knee is just proximal to the popliteal fossa, sit down. Press your knee into the client's hamstrings while you pull on her knee for an anterior leg stretch. Hold for a few seconds, then release.

Foot Press on the Urinary Bladder and Kidney Channels

Sit down at the client's feet. Flex her knee and hip. Hold her ankle in both hands. Press your inside foot as a "Mother foot" against the client's ischial tuberosity, then press your outside foot against her posterior thigh (Urinary Bladder and Kidney

channels). Pull the client's leg into your pressing foot. A push-pull action should occur at the same time (Fig. 9-9, *C*).

 ### CLIENT PRONE

Stomach and Spleen Channel Stretch

Kneel perpendicular to the client. Place a Mother-hand on her sacrum to stabilize. Grasp the client's foot with your other hand and flex her knee for a Stomach and Spleen Channel stretch. Hold for a few seconds, then release (Fig. 9-9, *D*).

Barefoot Shiatsu

Stand perpendicular to the client. Use the soles of your foot and toes to work her Urinary Bladder and Kidney Channels (Fig. 9-9, *E*).

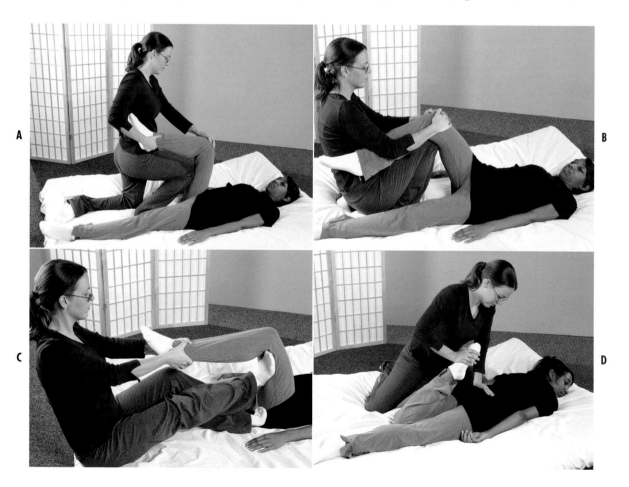

FIGURE 9-9 ▪ **A** and **B,** Knee on Urinary Bladder and Kidney Channels. **C,** Foot press on the posterior thigh. **D,** Stomach and Spleen Channel stretch.

Continued

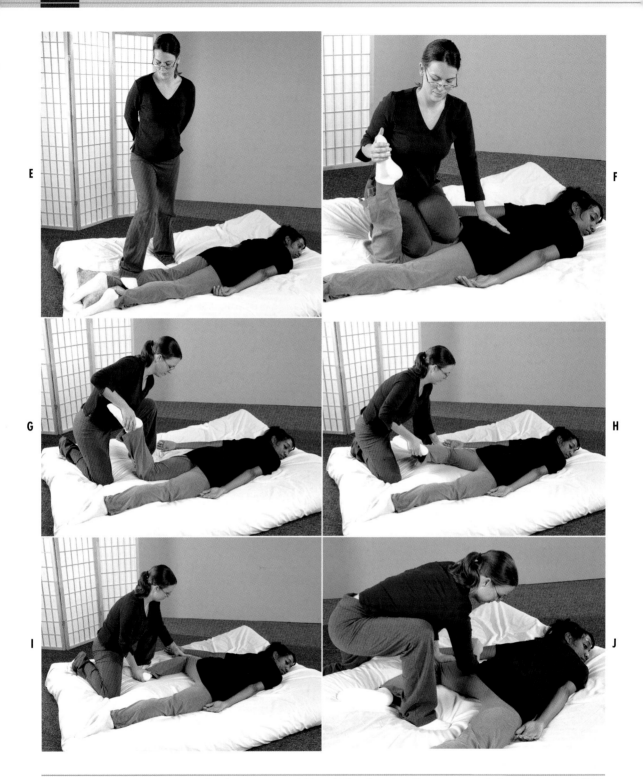

FIGURE 9-9, cont'd ■ **E,** Barefoot shiatsu on Urinary Bladder and Kidney Channels. **F,** Knees on posterior thigh. **G-J,** Forearm on Gallbladder Channel in frog stretch position.

Knees on Posterior Thigh

Sit perpendicular to the client; rest one or both of your knees (depending on the size of the client) on her posterior thigh. Place your Mother-hand on your client's sacrum or low back area. Grasp her foot with your other hand and flex her knee (Fig. 9-9, *F*).

You may rest your knees on the client's gastrocnemius, but only if the client has a sturdy gastrocnemius.

Frog Stretch Position

To place the client in the frog stretch position, kneel on one knee next to her by her legs. Move the client's arm so that it is at a 45-degree angle from her body. With your inside hand on the client's ankle and your outside hand supporting under her knee, flex her knee and swing her leg out laterally into hip flexion. Move your body as you put the client in frog stretch position so that you end up as shown in the Figure 9-9, *G* to *J*. Palm, thumb, and use your forearm, elbow, and knee on Gallbladder Channel (Fig. 9-9, *G-J*).

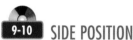

SIDE POSITION

Pin and Stretch Gallbladder Channel

Kneel next to the client's back, facing her head. Place your outside hand on the client's shoulder. Stretch her shoulder while pinning Gallbladder at her occiput with the thumb of your inside hand (Fig. 9-10, *A*).

Bilateral Forearm Stretch on the Torso

Kneel perpendicular to the client at her back. Place one forearm just inferior to the client's axilla and the other forearm just superior to her iliac crest. Lean forward and stretch outward along the client's torso. Hold for a few seconds, then release (Gallbladder Channel) (Fig. 9-10, *B*).

KNEE ON GALLBLADDER CHANNEL

Kneel perpendicular to the client's upper leg. Rest one hand on her knee and your other hand on her ankle. Use your knee on the client's Gallbladder Channel in her leg and lower leg (Fig. 9-10, *C*).

BAREFOOT SHIATSU

Stand perpendicular to the client. Press Gallbladder Channel with the soles of your feet and your toes (Fig. 9-10, *D*).

FULL LEG STRETCH

Sit at the client's feet. With her lower leg flexed at the knee joint, place the soles of both your feet against the client's shin. Grasp the ankle of her stretched-out upper leg with both hands. Push against the client's shin while pulling her stretched-out leg. Hold for a few seconds, then release (Fig. 9-10, *E*).

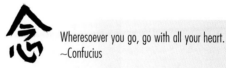

Wheresoever you go, go with all your heart.
~Confucius

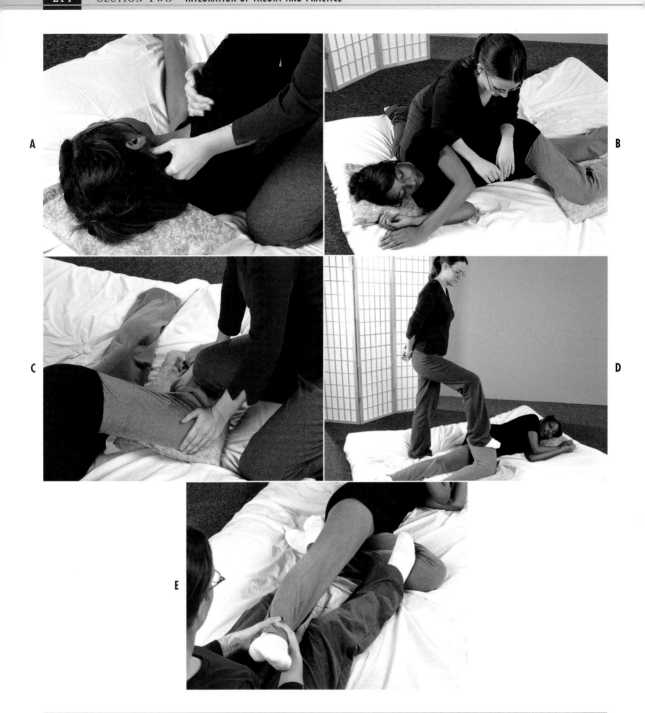

FIGURE 9-10 ■ **A,** Pin and stretch Gallbladder Channel. **B,** Bilateral forearm stretch on torso. **C,** Knee on Gallbladder Channel. **D,** Barefoot shiatsu on Gallbladder Channel. **E,** Full leg stretch.

1. Practice, practice, practice! Practice and integrate all the techniques shown in this chapter into shiatsu treatments until your own creative style of shiatsu emerges. See which of the techniques work for you and which do not. Create your own techniques. Most of all, enjoy yourself! Practice on at least two clients a week. These practice sessions should be documented and include the following:

    • Recipient's name
    • Recipient's age
    • Results of the pretreatment interview with the recipient
    • What channel was jitsu and what channel was kyo in the hara assessment
    • Results from all the other assessments you performed
    • Incorporation of specific channel work into the treatment: what channels you addressed and the techniques you used on those channels
    • How you addressed other areas of kyo and jitsu on the recipient
    • Any other techniques you used
    • How the recipient responded to the techniques you used
    • Pertinent information from the posttreatment discussion
    • Recommendations you gave the recipient for self-care

CONCEPTION VESSEL AND GOVERNING VESSEL

Conception (Directing) Vessel and Governing Vessel belong to the Eight Extraordinary Vessels and thus are not included in the 12 organ channels. They are mentioned in the Qigong section in Chapter 5.

Conception Vessel and Governing Vessel are two strong currents of energy that have wide-reaching functions and effects in the body. Both are located in the midline of the body; Conception Vessel travels up the anterior midline and Governing Vessel travels up the posterior midline. This relation to the core of the body is an indication of how powerful these vessels are.

Because Conception Vessel and Governing Vessel are part of the Eight Extraordinary Vessels, they usually are not addressed during a shiatsu session, except incidentally as the practitioner is working the primary channels. However, resting the Mother-hand on either Conception Vessel or Governing Vessel connects the central circulation of Ki to the channel being worked. Further study of these vessels is encouraged for the student interested in incorporating them more specifically into shiatsu treatments.

CONCEPTION (DIRECTING) VESSEL

The Chinese name for Conception Vessel is *Ren Mai.* Conception Vessel is the "Sea of Yin." The points on it nurture the Yin, Blood, and Essence of the body. Their purpose is to stabilize and descend Qi.

Conception Vessel arises in the lower abdomen and emerges in the center of the perineum. It travels up the front of the body, through the abdomen and chest, up through the anterior neck, and ends in the depression on the chin just below the lower lip (Fig. A-1).

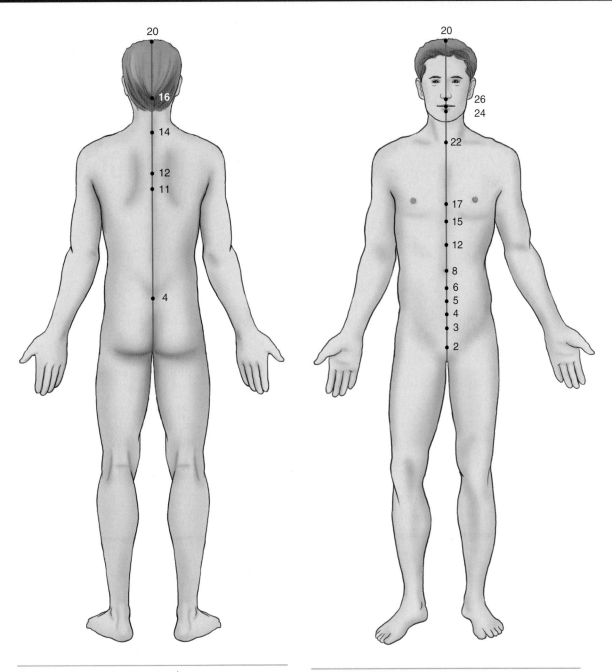

FIGURE A-1 ■ Conception Vessel.

FIGURE A-2 ■ Governing Vessel.

GOVERNING VESSEL

The Chinese name for Governing Vessel is *Du Mai*. Governing Vessel is the "Sea of Yang." The points on it invigorate the Yang, Source Qi, and Defensive Qi of the body. They also clear the mind. Their purpose is to sustain and raise Qi (Fig. A-2).

Governing Vessel originates in the lower abdomen and emerges in the center of the perineum. It travels up the back, over the top of the head, down the forehead and nose, and ends on a point that is one third the distance between the upper lip and nose.

BIBLIOGRAPHY

Anthony C: *A guide to the I Ching,* Stow, MA, 1988, Anthony Publishing Company.

Beinfield H, Korngold E: *Between heaven and earth,* New York, 1991, Ballantine.

Beresford-Cooke C: *Shiatsu theory and practice: a comprehensive text for the student professional,* ed 2, Philadelphia, 2003, Churchill Livingstone.

Connelly D: *Traditional acupuncture, the law of the Five Elements,* Columbia, MD, 1994, Traditional Acupuncture Institute.

Dubitsky C: *Bodywork shiatsu,* Rochester, VT, 1997, Healing Arts Press.

Ellis A, Feit R: *Fundamentals of Chinese acupuncture,* Brookline, MA, 1994, Paradigm Publications.

Endo R: *The new shiatsu method,* Tokyo, 2004, Kodansha International.

Ferguson P: *Take five, the Five Elements guide to health and harmony,* Dublin, 2000, Newleaf.

Gascoigne S: *Chinese way to health,* London, 1997, Eddison Sadd.

Hicks A, Hicks J, Mole P: *Five Element constitutional acupuncture,* Philadelphia, 2004, Churchill Livingstone.

Holland A: *Voices of Qi,* Seattle, WA, 1997, Northwest Institute of Acupuncture & Oriental Medicine.

Jackson C, Jackson J: *A study of shiatsu,* London, 2002, Caxton Editions.

Jarmey C, Mojay G: *Shiatsu: the complete guide,* London, 1999, Thorsons (HarperCollins).

Kaptchuk T: *The web that has no weaver,* Chicago, 2000, Contemporary Books.

Liechti E: *The complete illustrated guide to shiatsu,* Boston, 1998, Element Books.

Lundberg P: *The book of shiatsu,* New York, 2003, Simon and Schuster.

Maciocia G: *The foundations of Chinese medicine,* Philadelphia, 2005, Elsevier.

Masunaga S, Ohashi W: *Zen shiatsu,* Tokyo, 1997, Japan Publications.

Matsumoto K, Birch S: *Extraordinary Vessels,* Brookline, MA, 1986, Paradigm Publications.

Namikoshi T: *The complete book of shiatsu therapy,* Tokyo, 1981, Japan Publications.

Ohashi W: *Beyond shiatsu, Ohashi's bodywork method,* New York, 1996, Kodansha International.

Ohashi W: *The Ohashi bodywork book,* New York, 1996, Kodansha International.

Pritchard S: *Chinese massage manual: the healing art of tui na,* New York, 1999, Sterling Publishing.

Reichstein G: *Wood becomes water,* New York, 1998, Kodansha America.

Sergel D: *The natural way of zen shiatsu,* Tokyo, 1989, Japan Publications.

Serizawa K: *Tsubo: vital points for Oriental therapy,* Tokyo, 1976, Japan Publications.

Somma C: *Shiatsu,* New Jersey, 2007, Pearson Prentice Hall.

Yamamoto S: *Barefoot shiatsu,* Tokyo, 1979, Japan Publications.

Yanchi L, Zhanwen L, editors: *Basic theories of traditional Chinese medicine,* Beijing, 1995, Academy Press (Xue Yuan).

The Yellow Emperor's classic of internal medicine, Berkeley, CA, 2002, University of California (translated by I. Veith).

Ziyin S, Zelin C: *The basis of traditional Chinese medicine,* Boston, 1994, Shambhala.

GLOSSARY

Acupressure a technique based on the same principles as acupuncture. It involves the practitioner placing physical pressure with his or her palms, fingers, thumbs, or elbows on specific points along the channels of the body to release blocked Ki flow.

Acupuncture a technique involving the insertion and manipulation of needles into specific points on the body to release blocked Qi flow.

Ampuku deep abdominal massage.

Anma (Amma) the Japanese form of bodywork that developed from the Chinese Anmo; the precursor to shiatsu.

Anmo the Chinese form of bodywork that evolved from the ancient practice of An Wu. Its focus on musculoskeletal disorders and injuries laid the foundations for medical bone setting called Tuina.

An Wu one of the earliest forms of bodywork in China. It was developed more than 5000 years ago and resembles Western massage, using pressing, gliding, stretching, and percussing techniques on the body. The practitioner used his or her thumbs, fingers, forearms, elbows, knees, and feet on the points along the channels of Qi.

Asking one of the Four Methods of Assessment in traditional Chinese medicine. During the asking assessment the practitioner gets information from the client about how he or she is feeling and any conditions that may influence the design of the shiatsu treatment. It also establishes a connection between the practitioner and the client. The asking assessment consists of two parts: an intake form (pretreatment form or health history form) and a pretreatment session interview.

Assisted Fire (Lesser Fire, Supplemental Fire) one of the Five Elements. Associated with Fire, its correspondences are the same as for Fire. Its Yin organ and channel is Heart Protector; its Yang organ and channel is Triple Heater.

Assisted Fire (Lesser Fire, Supplemental Fire) Makka-ho a stretch developed by Makka specifically for the Heart Protector and Triple Heater channels.

Bad Diet eating foods that are processed, overeating one particular type of food, eating under stress or because of stress, and eating too quickly; all can contribute to illness in the body. In particular, overeating foods that are cold, raw, sweet, and high in fat can injure the Spleen and Stomach.

Basic Kata a routine that allows students to learn and reinforce elementary movements and proper body mechanics of shiatsu.

Blood in traditional Chinese medicine, it is the actual physical substance as well as a liquid form of Yin. It nourishes body tissues and organs; is cooling, soothing, and hydrating; and has an emotional and spiritual attachment. It is the responsibility of Blood to soothe, calm, and provide respite for the Shen.

Body Fluids the most Yin of all body substances, they are supported by Kidney Yin. The Body Fluids include cerebrospinal fluid, synovial fluid, serous fluid, mucus, urine, tears, sweat, lymph, and blood. Blood, however, is so important that it is considered in its own domain.

Body Mechanics the stance and movements a practitioner uses during a bodywork treatment to reduce the risk of injury to himself or herself and to perform as effective and efficient a treatment as possible.

Center of Gravity the axial core, physically and energetically, of the practitioner's body; the weight-balance point from superior to inferior and from side to side.

Channels (Meridians) streams of Ki flow located in specific areas of the body. Channels are connected to the organs of the body; the Ki in the channels is the living force that causes the organs to function.

Cold a contracting and freezing force. Ki slows and possibly stops moving, which causes pain. The body's metabolism slows down, and the body becomes underactive. The person craves warmth and has chills and shivering. Examples of Cold invasion are cold hands and feet, abdominal pain, pain and contraction of tendons, and aversion to cold. The person has a desire for warmth and warm drinks and foods. Examples of extreme Cold invasion are hypothermia and frostbite. The main organs and channels affected by Cold are the Bladder and Kidneys.

Coming from the Hara the fusion of relaxed body, centered mind, unrestricted breathing, free flow of Ki, stability, and powerful connection to the earth. The practitioner uses his or her hara as the source of Ki and strength needed to form a Ki connection with a client to perform as effective and efficient a shiatsu treatment as possible.

Completing the Circuit the placement of the practitioner's Mother-hand and Son-hand on the client so the practitioner's Ki can support the client's Ki. The Mother-hand connects with and receives input about the client's Ki. The Ki connection travels through the practitioner, and the practitioner's Ki supports the client's Ki. This reinforced Ki connection travels down through the practitioner's other arm and out through the Son-hand.

Conception (Directing) Vessel (Ren Mai) arises in the lower abdomen and emerges in the center of the perineum, then travels up the midline of the anterior body; called the "Sea of Yin." Its points nurture the Yin, Blood, and Essence of the body and stabilize and descend Ki.

Connection the therapeutic bond that forms between the practitioner and the client.

Constitution a person's physical makeup; determined by genetic factors, prenatal care, nutrition, and events surrounding birth.

Control Cycle the diagram that shows that each element actively controls another. This compensatory mechanism exists to restrain imbalances in the Creation Cycle. Earth controls Water; earthen dams keep water in check. Metal controls Wood; metal can cut through wood. Water controls Fire; water puts fire out. Wood controls Earth; trees are planted to prevent soil erosion, and plant roots can break through Earth and rock. Fire controls Metal; fire heats metal so it can be shaped.

Creation Cycle (Generation, Promoting, or Nurturing Cycle)   the circle of each element supporting, developing, and nourishing the element that follows it, much as a mother nourishes a child. Earth supports Metal; metals form within the earth. Metal supports Water; metals are minerals and leach into springs. Water supports Wood; trees need water to grow. Wood supports Fire; wood is fuel for fire. Fire supports Earth; the ashes from fire fortify the soil, and earth is made from cooled magma.

Damp   state of being wet, heavy, slow, and turbid; can be caused by external factors such as living in a damp house or damp weather. The main characteristics of Dampness in the body are heaviness in the head and body, stickiness, conditions that are difficult to get rid of, and repeated attacks of symptoms. It lingers and descends in the body, causing joint problems, swelling, fullness in the chest and abdomen, diarrhea, and fatigue. The organs and channels affected by damp are Stomach and Spleen. When Exterior Damp invades the body, it invades the legs first then moves upward through the leg channels and may settle in the pelvis. If this happens, it may endanger the reproductive organs.

Damp-Cold   state of being wet, heavy, slow, and turbid; can obstruct the Lungs, such as in bronchitis.

Damp-Heat   state of being wet, heavy, slow, and turbid; can appear as a vaginal infection or prostate inflammation accompanied by fever. It is most frequent in summer and late summer.

Dan Tien   located approximately three fingers' width inferior to two fingers' width behind the navel; it is the center of the practitioner's Qi. The practitioner must concentrate to generate his or her Qi from here. The Dan Tien is important in Qigong, martial arts, and Asian bodywork therapies. The lower Dan Tien (at the navel) is associated with physical energy and sometimes sexuality. The middle Dan Tien (at the solar plexus) deals with respiration and the health of internal organs. The upper Dan Tien (at the third eye) relates to consciousness, or Shen, and the brain.

Defensive Qi (Wei Qi)   a highly active Qi that protects the body from external pathogens and other harmful influences from the external environment. It is sent out by the Lungs and flows more toward the surface of the body (between muscles and the skin).

Do-In (Tao-Yinn)   a practice similar to yoga. It is a combination of exercises for channel stretching, breathing, Qi flow, and self-massage.

Dryness   a Yang pathogenic factor that tends to injure Yin or Blood; can be caused by a dry environment, dry wind, or dry indoor heating. It dries the mucous membranes and causes thirst and constipation. The main organs and channels affected by Dryness are the Lungs and Large Intestine.

Earth   one of the Five Elements. Its correspondences include the season of late summer, the color yellow, the development stage of transformation, the sense organ the mouth, and the emotion pensiveness. Its Yin organ and channel is Spleen; its Yang organ and channel is Stomach.

Earth Makka-Ho   a stretch developed by Makka specifically for the Stomach and Spleen Channels.

Essence (Jing)   the foundation of the body's physical structure. Three types of Essence exist: Prenatal Essence, Postnatal Essence, and Kidney Essence.

Excess Sexual Activity   an amount different for each person. Factors include age, constitution, and amount of sexual activity. For men, ejaculation is a loss of Essence. Women tend not to lose as much Essence during sex. However, both men and women can deplete the Kidneys through too many orgasms. If recovery time is not adequate, Essence and the Kidneys are not able to rejuvenate their Qi.

External Causes of Disease (Pernicious Influences or Weather)   outside influences that can challenge the body. These causes include Wind, Cold, Heat, Summer Heat, Damp, and Dryness and can cause similar conditions internally.

Fire one of the Five Elements. Its correspondences include the season of summer, the color red, the development stage of growth, the sense organ the tongue, and the emotion joy. Its Yin organ and channel is Heart; its Yang organ and channel is Small Intestine. Also associated with Fire is Assisted Fire (Lesser Fire, Supplemental Fire). Assisted Fire has the same correspondences as Fire; the assisted Fire Yin organ and channel is Heart Protector; the Yang organ and channel is Triple Heater.

Fire Makka-Ho a stretch developed by Makka specifically for the Heart and Small Intestine Channels.

Five Element Shiatsu a type of shiatsu that focuses on patterns of disharmony in the Five Element cycle as an assessment tool. The treatment plan uses techniques to balance the client's Ki and restore the harmony of the Five Element cycle.

Five Elements (Five Phases, Five Transformations) the traditional Chinese medicine method of ordering of the Qi of the universe into five different concepts: Wood, Fire, Earth, Metal, and Water. Each of the elements has corresponding Yin and Yang organs and channels.

Fixed Tsubo classic tsubo; their locations and effects have been studied and recorded for thousands of years. Their locations are set and found in virtually the same spot on every person. The Ki related to the functions of the organs and metabolic processes connect with universal Ki through the fixed tsubo.

Focus the practitioner's ability to concentrate on and attend to the client's therapeutic needs.

The Four Methods assessment methods used in traditional Chinese medicine: listening, observing, palpating, and asking.

Gallbladder the Yang organ and channel of the Wood element. Its functions in the human body include controlling digestive secretions and distributing emotional and physical Ki. It is related to the eyes and tendons, flexibility, clarity in everyday decision making, and the ability to take risks versus timidity. It symbolically represents accomplishment and courage; in traditional Chinese medicine it stores and excretes bile and controls judgment and decision making.

Governing Vessel (Du Mai) originates in the lower abdomen and emerges in the center of the perineum, then travels up the midline of the posterior body; it is the "Sea of Yang." Its points invigorate the Yang, Source Qi, and defensive Qi of the body; clear the mind; and sustain and raise Qi.

Hara abdominal area or belly; it is also the core of the body. It is the source of the shiatsu practitioner's Ki. The hara is also where Ki can usually most easily be palpated on a client.

Hara Assessment a part of the palpation assessment; a specific routine the practitioner uses in touching the client's belly to assess kyo and jitsu in each of the channels to gain information about the state of the client's Ki.

Hara Headlights the act of the practitioner having his or her hara facing the area of the client's body being worked on; the practitioner's hara shines on that part of the client's body.

Heart the Yin organ and channel of the Fire Element. Its function in the body includes adaptation and the emotional interpretation of experience. It is related to the heart, tongue, speech, and the brain. It symbolically represents emotional adaptation, emotional stability, and spirit. In traditional Chinese medicine it governs and propels the blood and controls the blood vessels.

Heart Protector (Heart Constrictor, Pericardium) the Yin organ and channel of Assisted Fire. Its function in the body includes being the minister to the Heart, protecting Shen, providing circulation for the inner core, and governing the vascular system. It is related to the heart, blood vessels, and circulation; it symbolically represents emotional stability, protection of the blood and defense of the emotional core. In traditional Chinese medicine it maintains consciousness by a connection with Source Qi, Heart, and Shen. It is an energetic buffer zone around the heart, protecting it and the blood of the heart. It is related to circulation of blood in the great vessels and ensures the stability of Shen.

Heat   the body feels hot, and a fever can be present. It often occurs in summer but can be present in other seasons as well. The fluids concentrate and become yellow, and sweating occurs. Heat creates more thirst and sweat. Movement of Qi speeds up, but it is restless movement. Localized Heat can be caused by localized infections characterized by redness, pain, heat, and swelling. The main organs and channels affected by Heat are Heart, Heart Protector, Small Intestine, and Triple Heater.

Herbal Therapy   a traditional medicine based on the use of plants and plant extracts.

Incorrect Treatment   the wrong treatment for a particular condition. Incorrect treatment can happen in any type of treatment, Eastern or Western, throughout the world. If a person's condition is treated incorrectly, the original problem is not solved and it may lead to worse ones.

Internal Causes of Disease (Emotions)   mental and/or emotional issues that can cause disease according to traditional Chinese medicine. These causes include joy, worry, sadness (and grief), anger, fear, and severe fright (shock).

Internal Cold   a contracting and freezing force caused by Yang deficiency. It can also be caused by overeating iced foods and drinks.

Internal Dampness   condition of being wet, heavy, slow, and turbid; generated by a weak Spleen and sometimes Kidneys. Clinical manifestations develop gradually rather than suddenly. Lack of exercise, which slows the Qi, can be a cause. Diet plays a significant role in dampness. Old, cold food (such as leftovers), canned food, foods high in fat, dairy products, excessive meat intake, and fried foods all create Dampness.

Internal Dryness   comes from Yin deficiency of the Stomach and/or Kidneys. Because the Stomach is the origin of fluids, eating late at night, following an irregular diet, or becoming active too quickly after eating can deplete Stomach fluids and increase dryness in the body.

Internal Heat   can result from any issue involving Qi stagnation. As the Qi stagnates, it creates Heat. Heat also occurs from living in a hot climate and overeating hot foods.

Internal Wind   starts with a Liver problem and can gradually develop into tremors, seizures, stroke, or Alzheimer's disease.

Intuition   the ability of a practitioner to piece together many small bits of information from and about a client until a complete picture of the client's therapeutic needs is formed.

Jitsu   areas of the body that are full or have excessive Ki.

Kanji   the Japanese writing system that uses characters adapted from Chinese letters.

Kata   a routine used in martial arts to help students learn moves and techniques in a logical sequence. Information is presented in such a way that every step builds on previously acquired knowledge. It is also used in bodywork such as shiatsu.

Key Classic Tsubo   tsubo (or points) that, when addressed through shiatsu, acupuncture, or moxibustion, can alleviate particular conditions.

Ki (Qi)   the energy or force that gives and maintains life and the connection between organisms and all of creation. The Chinese spelling is Qi, and the Japanese spelling is Ki. In the body, Ki is the source behind the substances and structures as well as the energy and movement of substances and structures. It flows in specific channels connected to the organs of the body.

Ki Connection   the therapeutic bond that forms between the practitioner and the client as each one's Ki meets and supports the other.

Ki Patterns   a part of the observing assessment; part of how the client's Ki is presenting in his or her body: up or down, strong or weak, one side more than the other, spiraling, and/or flowing or blocked in certain areas.

Kidney refers to the Yin organ and channel of the Water element. Its function in the body includes water metabolism and governance of the endocrine system. It is related to the kidneys, pituitary and adrenal glands, stress response, sexual hormones and the desire for reproduction, the ears, and bones. It symbolically represents impetus, flexibility, and the ability to respond to a stimulus. In traditional Chinese medicine it houses the Essence, stores fundamental Yin and Yang of the body, governs water, grasps or anchors Lung Ki, produces the brain and the central nervous system, and houses willpower and ambition.

Kidney Essence supports the Yin of the entire being. Both Prenatal and Postnatal Essence is part of Kidney Essence, which circulates throughout the body.

Kyo areas of the body that are empty or deficient in Ki.

Large Intestine the Yang organ and channel of the Metal element. Its function in the body is elimination; it is related to the large intestine, mouth, throat, and bowel movements. It symbolically represents the ability to release, and in traditional Chinese medicine it descends its Ki and allows passage of waste.

Listening one of the Four Methods of Assessment in traditional Chinese medicine. During the listening assessment, the practitioner listens to what the client is saying, how he or she is saying it, and perhaps what the client is not saying. Although what the client is saying is important, the practitioner can also open his or her awareness to the tone and timbre of the client's voice.

Liver the Yin organ and channel of the Wood element. Its functions in the body include storing nutrients, controlling the free flow of Ki throughout the body, governing detoxification, and controlling the blood. It is related to detoxification, vision, the eyes,

tendons, energetic and emotional ups and downs, and major decision making. It symbolically represents choice and the execution of one's life plan, vision, planning, and action. In traditional Chinese medicine it gives the capacity for being goal oriented and resolute, ensures the smooth flow of Ki, and stores the Blood.

Lung the Yin organ and channel of the Metal element. Its function in the body is the intake of Ki; it is related to the nose, lungs, and skin. It symbolically represents boundaries. In traditional Chinese medicine it governs Ki, disperses fluids and Wei Qi, descends the Ki, and regulates water passages.

Macrobiotic (Barefoot) Shiatsu developed by Shizuko Yamamoto, this practice mingles macrobiotic nutritional principles with shiatsu techniques. This style of shiatsu combines pressure on tsubo with stretches and physical manipulation. It is called barefoot Shiatsu because practitioners originally used their bare feet to apply many techniques. Currently, barefoot Shiatsu refers to techniques specifically applied with the feet, whether bare or wearing socks.

Makka-ho (Makka's method, Makka's exercises) a series of stretches based on the channel pairs developed by Makka in the 1970s. They serve as a reminder for channel locations, provide an overall stretch to every area of the body, and can bring to the shiatsu practitioner awareness of imbalances in his or her own body.

Meditation the act of engaging in mental and physical exercise for the purpose of reaching a heightened level of spiritual awareness.

Metal one of the Five Elements; its correspondences include the season of autumn, the color white, the development stage of harvest, the sense organ of the nose, and the emotions sadness and grief. Its Yin organ and channel is Lung; its Yang organ and channel is Large Intestine.

Metal Makka-Ho a stretch developed by Makka specifically for the Lung and Large Intestine Channels.

Mother-hand the shiatsu practitioner's hand that remains stationary on the client; it usually is placed near the client's hara and acts as an instrument of baseline measurement of the client's Ki.

Moxibustion techniques involving the application of herbal heat to specific points on the body. Moxa (mugwort herb) is aged, then ground into a fluff or processed further into a stick shape that resembles a cigar. It can be used indirectly, as with acupuncture needles, or burned directly on the skin.

Namikoshi (Nippon) Shiatsu a common type of shiatsu in Japan developed by Tokujiro Namikoshi. It involves a whole body routine that incorporates stretches, but the emphasis is more on addressing points (tsubo) than channels. It tends to be a vigorous treatment.

Nonfixed Tsubo tsubo that can occur anywhere along a channel; they reveal the ever-changing Ki flow and manifest as tangible, palpable points that are jitsu or kyo.

Observing one of the Four Methods of Assessment in traditional Chinese medicine. During the observing assessment, the practitioner assesses the client for visual clues. The shiatsu practitioner can use three main categories of observation: hue of the client's face; the client's posture, body movements, and demeanor; and the client's body energy patterns.

Ohashiatsu a type of shiatsu developed by Wataru Ohashi, who opened the Shiatsu Institute in New York City in 1974. Ohashiatsu focuses less on finger pressure along the channels and more on stretching and physically manipulating the client's body to achieve Ki balance.

Organs in traditional Chinese medicine, organs have specific physiologic functions similar to the functions of organs in Western science as well as emotional and spiritual correlations. The organs in traditional Chinese medicine are divided into Yin and Yang pairs and include Lung, Large Intestine, Stomach, Spleen, Heart, Small Intestine, Kidneys, Urinary Bladder, Liver, Gallbladder, Triple Heater, and Heart Protector. The channels connected to the organs have the same names: Lung Channel, Large Intestine Channel, and so forth.

Overexertion excess activity, whether mental, physical, or both; depletes Spleen Qi and Kidney Qi. If recovery time is not adequate, these two organs are not able to replenish their Qi and a systemic illness may occur.

Palpating one of the Four Methods of Assessment in traditional Chinese medicine. During the palpation assessment, the practitioner assesses the client by touch.

Parasites creatures that drain the body's resources and make the person vulnerable to illness; include athlete's foot, malaria, and hookworm.

Point See *tsubo*.

Poisons elements that drain the body's resources and make the person vulnerable to illness; they come from a variety of sources, including ingested chemicals, pollutants, and radiation.

Postnatal (Acquired) Essence produced from food by the Spleen and Stomach. It travels to all other parts of the body to support them as well as to the Kidneys, where it is stored. A healthy diet and physical fitness (to strengthen the body and provide good breathing) can contribute to the formation of Postnatal Essence, and a temperate lifestyle can preserve it.

Postural Patterns a part of the observing assessment; they are part of how a person carries himself or herself. Different types of posture can be caused by skeletal issues, muscle tension, injury, and trauma and can manifest as certain areas as being kyo and jitsu.

Prenatal (Congenital) Essence responsible for the genetic physical constitution of the body; it is present from conception and stored between the Kidneys.

Qi see *Ki*.

Qigong means "energy cultivation." It is an aspect of traditional Chinese medicine involving the coordination of different breathing patterns with various physical postures and motions of the body. It is mostly taught for maintaining health but can also be used therapeutically and in martial arts.

Self-Care practices that maintain health, such as a balanced diet, proper water intake, and enough sleep.

Self Check-in the process of a practitioner performing a mental body scan on himself or herself to let go of muscle tension and non-treatment-related thoughts and remain centered and grounded while using proper body mechanics.

Shen most closely translated as the mind and/or spirit. It is the most metaphysical of the Vital Substances. Because the body cannot live without the mind or the spirit, it is inextricably linked to the corporeal being and therefore linked to Qi and Essence. Shen gives the person his or her sense of self, also known as consciousness.

Shiatsu a Japanese form of bodywork. Its name comes from the Japanese words *shi,* meaning finger, and *atsu,* meaning pressure. It is a hands-on therapy based on the same principles as acupuncture—that Ki flows in channels throughout the person. When pain or discomfort is present, the Ki flow is disrupted in some way. During treatment the client remains fully clothed while the shiatsu practitioner applies his or her palms, fingers, thumbs, forearms, elbows, knees, feet, and toes to the client's body and uses stretches and range-of-motion techniques to rebalance the client's Ki flow and alleviate the pain or discomfort.

Small Intestine the Yang organ and channel of the Fire Element. Its function in the body is assimilation and absorption of food and experiences of all kinds; it is related to the small intestine, the spine, cerebrospinal fluid, and the body's mechanisms for dealing with shock. It symbolically represents assimilation, being filled and transforming. In traditional Chinese medicine it separates the pure from the impure.

Son-Hand the shiatsu practitioner's hand that moves along the client's channels, assessing the client's Ki by comparing it to the Ki felt by the Mother-hand. The Son-hand is also used to free blockages of Ki, bring Ki to areas that are deficient, and disperse areas that have too much Ki.

Source Qi the Yang expression of Qi, it is the basic form of Qi in the body composed of a combination of the essential Qi of the Kidney; Qi of food, derived through the transformative function of the Spleen; and air (Great Qi), drawn in through the Lungs. Source Qi serves to energize all the organs, including the organs that helped create it, and is the basis of all physical activity. It is the energy of movement and transformation. All forms of Qi in the body are derivatives of Source Qi.

Spleen the Yin organ and channel of the Earth element. Its function in the body is digestive secretions; it is related to thinking, pancreatic enzymes, stomach and small intestine juices, and the hormones insulin and glucagon. It symbolically represents nurturing, fertility, digestion of food and ideas, and the ability to think and learn. In traditional Chinese medicine it contains the blood, controls the muscles, lifts the Ki, and houses thought.

Stomach refers to the Yang organ and channel of the Earth element. Its functions in the body include intake of food and transportation of nutrients to the digestive tract. It is related to the digestive tract, appetite, ovaries, the uterus, and the menstrual cycle. It symbolically represents nurturing, fertility, and groundedness. In traditional Chinese medicine it controls the rotting and ripening of food.

Summer Heat only occurs in summer; the main symptoms are headache, aversion to heat, sweating, thirst, and dark and scanty urine. Summer Heat may also cause hyperthermia such as heat cramps, heat stroke, and heat exhaustion. The organs and channels affected by Heat are Heart, Heart

Protector, Small Intestine, and Triple Heater.

Tao   a term translated to mean road, path, way, means, doctrine, God, the universe, nature, that which is, the way, or the path. The Tao is the primary law of the universe, the law that is the genesis for all other laws and principles of the workings of the universe and the world.

Tensegrity   a term coined by architect, engineer, and scientist R. Buckminster Fuller. The basic principles of tensegrity are that, in a stable system, a kind of push-pull relation exists. If a stress is placed on one part of the system, a change is caused (push) that is compensated for by another part of the system (pull). This ensures the stability of the system. If the compensation does not occur, or if the stress is greater than the compensation, the system could break down.

Three Treasures   the hara (center of the body), the point of one hundred meetings (on the top of the head; it pulls the body upward and keeps the back and posture straight), and bubbling spring (Kidney 1 on the bottom of the foot; it keeps the body grounded into the center of the earth).

Touch Sensitivity   the ability of a practitioner, by using his or her fingers, to detect subtle physical and energetic nuances in the tissues of a client's body.

Traditional Chinese Medicine   a variety of medical practices used in China that developed over several thousand years. It includes herbal medicine, acupuncture, and bodywork. Based on the theory that the processes of the human body are interconnected with the earth, discomfort and illness are regarded as disharmonies of a person's internal and/or external environment and should be treating accordingly.

Trauma   physical, mental, and emotional injury, stress, or shock; can cause stagnation of Qi and Blood. The stagnation can manifest in different organs and tissues, such as chronic headaches, tight muscles, and digestive disorders that in some cases can be quite painful. Even though traumas can heal, many years later the person can be vulnerable to other pernicious influences.

Triple Heater (San Jiao, Triple Burner, Triple Warmer)   the Yang organ and channel of Assisted Fire. Its functions in the body include psychologic protection, peripheral circulation of blood and lymph, and distribution of Source Qi and information among all organ systems. It is related to blood circulation, the lymphatic system, immunity, metabolism, allergic reactions, and stiff neck and shoulders. It symbolically represents protection versus openness, the body's surface, and defense against pathogens or emotional insult. In traditional Chinese medicine it is an avenue of distribution of Original Qi and has three spaces in the body that need to be warm and allow for transformation: upper burner (Lungs and Heart); middle burner (Stomach and Spleen); lower burner (Kidney, Urinary Bladder, Small Intestine and Large Intestine).

Tsubo (Point)   an opening or gateway into a channel and a direct link between the channels and the outside world. It is a place where Ki can be changed, dispersed, or supported through thumb or finger pressure or, in the case of acupuncture, through the insertion of a needle.

Tsubo Therapy   The stimulation of tsubo, whether through moxibustion, acupuncture, or finger pressure, to release blocked Ki flow.

Tuina   a form of Chinese bodywork that developed from Anmo. With the use of traditional Chinese medicine principles, the techniques include brushing, kneading, rolling, pressing, and rubbing the areas between each of the joints to get Qi moving in the channels and the muscles.

Underexertion   lack of physical activity and mental activity that causes a decrease in the circulation of Qi. It weakens the function of the Spleen and Stomach and decreases the body's resistance to disease.

Urinary Bladder   the Yang organ and channel of the Water element. Its functions in the body include governing the autonomic nervous system, transforming fluids, and purifying Ki. It is related to determination, intensity, fatigue, fear, the urinary bladder, the spine, bones, fluid balance, and reproduction. It symbolically represents impetus, the ability to respond, and fluidity. In traditional Chinese medicine it tones all the organ functions, receives impure fluids from the kidneys and transforms them, stores and excretes urine, and influences posture by giving strength and support to the back.

Vital Substances elements that embody all aspects of the body's structure and function; the physiologic and metabolic aspects of the body are considered as relations and interactions among vital substances. The vital substances are Ki, Blood, Essence, and Body Fluids.

Water one of the Five Elements. Its correspondences include the season of winter, the colors black or blue, the development stage of storage, the sense organ of the ears, and the emotion fear. Its Yin organ and channel is Kidney; its Yang organ and channel is Urinary Bladder.

Water Makka-Ho a stretch developed by Makka specifically for the Kidney and Urinary Bladder Channels.

Weak Constitution a diminished physical body and depleted Source Qi. It can be caused by illnesses, trauma, or genetics. If a person has a weak constitution, he or she is more susceptible to pernicious influences and illnesses.

Wind can be from the atmosphere or artificial wind pathogens such as fans, air conditioning, and open car windows. Wind creates movement in the body where stillness should be; even the symptoms of Wind can move within the body. Wind is the forerunner of other pernicious influences, and it usually teams up with the others to create Wind-Cold, Wind-Heat or Wind-Damp. The main organs and channels affected by Wind are Liver and Gallbladder.

Wind-Cold has a sudden onset and usually is a common cold or flu. Early symptoms include fatigue and headache that can develop into a mild fever; stuffy nose with a runny, clear discharge; body aches; and cough. Chills are also present. Sometimes Wind-Cold transforms into Wind-Heat.

Wind-Damp a state of being wet, heavy, slow, and turbid; has as its main symptoms itchy skin, urticaria, sweating, body aches, feeling of heaviness, and swollen joints. It is similar to Wind-Heat in that it manifests as stomach distress or nausea. However, it can penetrate the joints and develop into arthritis. It also can cause muscle aches and soreness that travel around the body.

Wind-Heat has a sudden onset with a fever. Symptoms include a stuffy nose with a yellow, sticky discharge; some body aches; an extremely sore throat; cough; headache; and fatigue. These are all classic signs of the flu.

Wood one of the Five Elements. Its correspondences include the season of spring, the color green, the development stage of birth, the sense organ of the eyes, and the emotion anger. Its Yin organ and channel is Liver; its Yang organ and channel is Gallbladder.

Wood Makka-Ho a stretch developed by Makka specifically for the Liver and Gallbladder channels.

Yellow Emperor's Classic of Internal Medicine (Huang Ti Nei Ching) a series of texts written during the Han Dynasty (206 BC-220 AD) that contain the fundamentals of all branches of Chinese medicine. Chinese physicians today still practice the theories explained in this text. It is written in the form of a dialogue in which the emperor seeks information from his minister, Ch'I-Po, on all questions relating to health and the art of healing.

Yin and Yang ancient Chinese philosophical concepts that describe two opposing but complementary forces, arising from the Tao, found in everything in the universe. They are not absolutes; instead, a continuum or relationship exists; one is flowing into the other, always transforming each other. They are the natural limits for each other; Yin can only go so far before it becomes Yang; Yang can only go so far before it becomes Yin.

Zen Shiatsu   a treatment emphasis developed by Shizuto Masunago that concerns the Ki flow in the channels more than addressing tsubo. The practitioner's intuition and connection with the client's Ki are important. The treatment can be either gentle or vigorous.

INDEX